D0143296

Carol Bucciarelli, MEd, CADC

Addicted and Mentally Ill
Stories of Courage, Hope, and Empowerment

Pre-publication
REVIEWS,
COMMENTARIES,
EVALUATIONS . . .

"**A** helpful perspective with some useful recommendations for families as they come to terms with the mental illness and/or addiction of those dear to them."

Stanton E. Samenow, PhD
Clinical Psychologist,
Author of *Inside the Criminal Mind*

"**A** must read for dually diagnosed individuals, their families, and clinicians who lack expertise with this population. Many families of individuals who are dually diagnosed do not understand the complexity of the disorder and feel helpless in taking care of their loved ones. This book gives hope and provides some practical strategies that can help clients and their families."

Stephen N. Campbell, PhD
Associate Professor,
Clinical/Community Psychology,
Center for Psychological Studies,
Nova Southeastern University

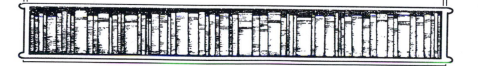

Addicted and Mentally Ill
Stories of Courage, Hope, and Empowerment

THE HAWORTH PRESS
Haworth Series in Family and Consumer Issues in Health
F. Bruce Carruth, PhD, Senior Editor

Addicted and Mentally Ill: Stories of Courage, Hope, and Empowerment by Carol Bucciarelli

Other Titles of Related Interest

Managing the Dually Diagnosed Patient: Current Issues and Clinical Approaches, Second Edition edited by David F. O'Connell and Eileen P. Beyer

Dual Disorders: Essentials for Assessment and Treatment by David F. O'Connell

Treating Co-Occurring Disorders: A Handbook for Mental Health and Substance Abuse Professionals by Edward L. Hendrickson, Marilyn S. Schmal, and Sharon C. Eckleberry

Designing, Implementing, and Managing Co-Occurring Treatment Services for Individuals with Mental Health and Substance Use Disorders: Blueprints for Action by Edward L. Hendrickson

Responding to Physical and Sexual Abuse in Women with Alcohol and Other Drug and Mental Disorders: Program Building edited by Bonita M. Veysey and Colleen Clark

Addicted and Mentally Ill
Stories of Courage, Hope, and Empowerment

Carol Bucciarelli, MEd, CADC

The Haworth Press®
New York • London • Oxford

BP 53

The Haworth Press, Inc., 10 Alice Street, Binghamton, NY 13904-1580.

The vignettes in this book are fictional stories. Any resemblance to actual persons, living or dead, is entirely coincidental and unintentional.

Cover design by Jennifer M. Gaska.

Library of Congress Cataloging-in-Publication Data

Bucciarelli, Carol.
    Addicted and mentally ill : stories of courage, hope, and empowerment / Carol Bucciarelli.
        p. cm.
    Includes bibliographical references and index.
    ISBN 0-7890-1885-3 (hard : alk. paper)—ISBN 0-7890-1886-1 (soft : alk. paper)
    1. Dual diagnosis—Treatment. 2. Dual diagnosis—Patients—Rehabilitation. 3. Dual diagnosis—Patients—Family relationships. I. Title.

RC564.68.B835 2004
362.29'186—dc22
                                                                2003028213

7/12/06

CONTENTS

ABOUT THE AUTHOR

Carol Bucciarelli, MEd, CADC, was a high school English teacher in Florida for two years and in New Jersey for four years. For four years she taught remedial English classes at a New Jersey community college. In 1989, she began working at The MICA Club (initially as a secretary) where she first developed an interest in the struggles of dually diagnosed individuals. During that time Ms. Bucciarelli received the necessary education to become a Certified Alcohol and Drug Counselor in the state of New Jersey. Since receiving her CADC, she has worked as a Habilitation Counselor at The MICA Club for two years and later as an inpatient Addiction Counselor at a hospital-based dual-diagnosis unit in New Jersey for seven years. Presently, she is a case manager for an intensive outpatient program in addictions at a behavioral health facility in New Jersey.

Preface

What Is MICA?

In the state of New Jersey, where I live, MICA stands for mentally ill, chemically abusing. Now and then, I see a van with MICA written on the side, filled with individuals being ferried to and from appointments, and I often wonder how it feels to be classified in that vaguely accusatory tone.

Millions of people in the United States today are walking around with undiagnosed or unacknowledged dual-diagnosis symptoms. A person who is "dually diagnosed" has been diagnosed with both mental illness and substance addiction. In many cases, this individual will have been hospitalized at least one time for his or her mental illness. The person's addiction may or may not be acknowledged, but it can be recognized by his or her preoccupation with substances or processes that cause increasing life losses and decreasing quality of life.

In my treatment of dually diagnosed individuals, one of the first questions they generally ask is, "Did I cause my mental illness by drug use?" Another common question is, "Did I get addicted by self-medicating my mental illness?" When presented with these questions, I focus on explaining that, though we may never be able to determine the exact causes of both of these diseases, we do know ways to control them: employing relapse prevention skills, taking medications, attending self-help support groups such as Narcotics Anonymous (NA), Alcoholics Anonymous (AA), and the National Alliance for the Mentally Ill (NAMI), and more.

It is important for the person recovering from mental illness and addiction, and for his or her family, to focus on what can be done to promote wellness rather than on mistakes that may have been made in the past. As the length of stays in treatment centers continually decreases and brief therapy becomes a greater necessity, individuals addressing these dual-recovery issues must be encouraged to focus on what can be done *now* to promote an improved lifestyle.

My purpose in writing this book is to give people in recovery and their families some insights on what being dually diagnosed can mean to them and, further, on how co-occurring mental illness and addiction can be treated with a minimum amount of blame, shame, and poor decision making. My hope is that those who read this book will be able to identify and take encouragement from the positives that can exist throughout the healing process within the family system of the dually diagnosed person.

Addressing substance abuse may not be anywhere near the beginning of the list of priorities for those diagnosed with mental illness and addiction. As trust is built and the individuals are able to understand more about their problems, their families and support systems can hope that the individuals will become more aware of the negative effects of substance abuse on their quality of life. Even when these individuals remain sober, they may experience their lives as chaotic, filled with stressors that cause their mental illness symptoms to return. Reducing that chaos and providing answers, nurturing, and understanding are the tasks of the families and support systems of people with mental illness and addiction.

As I found when I first came to the field of dual-diagnosis counseling approximately fifteen years ago, this is a complex but rewarding task. For several years I worked with dually diagnosed people who were living at home and coming to a treatment setting daily, usually for around five hours per day. Some of these individuals had been treated in a hospital setting first, and some had undergone drug detoxification for a few days. Many came to us barely sober, but with a strong desire to learn how to improve the quality of their lives.

In this setting, I had the opportunity to see people grow in ability and understanding on a daily basis. They came to us by van from group homes, apartments, their parents' homes, and shelters. They came hoping they could get stabilized on their medications. They came hoping not to drink or to use drugs for just one more day. They came because they no longer had families who wanted to speak to or spend time with them. Often, they came fleeing from the madness that dogged their days and nights, wanting the structure we provided through outpatient treatment. Mostly, though, they came because they needed someone to talk to—someone who understood the confusion and frustration of living with co-occurring diseases. I quickly learned that I held many misconceptions about people who are mentally ill addicts. As I spoke to these individuals and got to know them, I began to understand what *powerlessness* means.

I initially worked for a program based on a psychosocial model that followed a holistic approach to treatment to empower mentally ill individuals with addiction to grasp their strengths as they learned to manage their illnesses and lead productive lives. Our purpose was to give these individuals a chance to achieve something, no matter how small, that could restore their pride in themselves. In a supervised setting, dually diagnosed individuals were able to learn ways of relating to themselves and to others in a nonthreatening manner. Some of this was accomplished through establishing a recovery-based newspaper, creating a consumer-run kitchen that made lunches for other consumers and staff, and providing opportunities for art projects and even video making. I was amazed at the courage shown by these individuals. Some who had previously been suicidal would prepare lunch for thirty other people while waiting for their antidepressant medications to take effect, and others with schizophrenia would write articles for the newspaper while struggling with voices inside their heads.

Over time, some of these individuals became able to enter transitional employment. Counselors remained available to help them as they readjusted to the work world, while attending the outpatient program a few hours a week as their home base. It was highly rewarding to watch these individuals move forward in this fashion, using what they had learned and showing pride in themselves and in their work.

Having experienced the fulfillment of seeing people progress in an outpatient setting, I felt I was now ready to move on to what I thought would be more intense, frontline work—inpatient treatment. I had once visited a local inpatient rehabilitation facility, when one of our dually diagnosed clients had been sent there after a relapse, and had been impressed by the work they did.

Now, seven years later, I think that one of the primary focuses in dual-diagnosis work should be consumer advocacy. After years of calling on families who would not come in, of trying to arrange housing in places that "do not take those people," of trying to obtain services for consumers who cannot get disability coverage despite severe mental illness—after all these years, I believe that some of the answers for dually diagnosed people have to come from a change of attitude in society.

It is my hope, as I present constructed stories about people with mental illness and addiction who have come through our dual-diagnosis unit, that other dually diagnosed individuals and their families will see that addiction is not a moral issue but a disease. It is also my hope that readers will begin to see mental illness in a different light.

Often the prevailing feeling people have over being diagnosed with a mental illness is, at the beginning, deep shame, which is only compounded when they experience shame for the behaviors they may have exhibited as a result of their addiction. What I have found, in my years of providing dual-diagnosis counseling, is that individuals with mental illness and addiction often feel disconnected from the human race, isolated, and they do not know how to reconnect because, for years, that isolation may have been something they chose in order to feel safe. Now, in recovery, it has become even more difficult for them to face the world, with no substance to cushion the unpredictability of life. This is particularly true of those who suffer the symptoms of a continually recurring or worsening mental illness.

"Do not leave until the miracle happens" is an old self-help program saying. I find this to be exemplified often in the lives of people who benefit the most from treatment. Regardless of what I or any other staff member does, the person has to be "there" for it, to bring hope and steadfastness to the situation, something I can feed but not create. Such hope lends itself ultimately to reconnecting the person with mental illness and addiction to all, or much, that he or she has lost.

Family members and support systems can aid in reestablishing that connection, no matter how tenuous. As you will see in the following vignettes, sometimes I was able to assist in helping these individuals reconnect, but sometimes my own frustration with a consumer or lack of knowledge got in the way. The people whom you will meet in these vignettes are constructed individuals whose situations are only representative of what goes on in a dual-diagnosis inpatient setting. In providing these fictional stories, I have attempted to convey the intensity and urgency of the dually diagnosed person's life experience as he or she seeks change and stabilization.

Acknowledgments

To all the dually diagnosed individuals with whom I have worked in the past several years, I give my thanks and respect. Your struggles and your victories have made a lasting impression on me, and I hope with this manuscript to impart this impression to others.

A special thanks goes to Joan Treske, who was my mentor as I learned about dual diagnosis. When working with Joan at the MICA Club, I watched as she prioritized even the smallest interactions with her dually diagnosed "members" of the club. What they had to say or do was the most important business of the day. Later, when I began working in an inpatient program and would be overwhelmed with daily tasks, I remembered what Joan had taught me: Focus only on that person waiting by your door. Be there for that person. Listen.

Finally, I owe a debt of gratitude to Dr. Bruce Carruth, who spent many months helping me edit this book. He, too, takes Joan's client-centered focus. His respect for and desire to help the dually diagnosed individual shines through his work and was a strong influence on me as I wrote and edited this book.

Chapter 1

Dual Diagnosis and the Family System

What is home to you? Is it a place where you can be yourself? Or is it a place where you have to "toe the line," always meeting the expectations of others? For dually diagnosed people, home often turns out to be a place where they are continually observed. Are they using drugs? Are they complying with their medication regimen? Is their behavior erratic?

People with mental illness and addiction, even when remaining sober, may see certain manifestations of their mental illness as a big part of who they are. People who suffer from rapid mood swings may feel more creative when they are in a "high" mood, whereas their families may experience this type of mood as grandiosity or the behavior as "overexcited" and lacking in judgment. What a family member calls "those voices in your head" may seem, to a dually diagnosed person, his or her own special kind of reality. At times, such a person may have periodic needs to isolate, or fears that appear to make sense to no one but himself or herself. Though prescribed medication can alleviate or reduce mental illness symptoms, individuals may refuse or cut down on medications that make them feel unlike themselves. At times, recovering people may feel very much like themselves, but, to others, they may appear unstable.

From the family's point of view (whether family consists of the dually diagnosed person's parents, children, or significant others), living with someone whose behavior is not always consistent is both frightening and unnerving. Families may become oversensitive or even defensive about behaviors that are not symptoms of mental illness simply because they are so fearful of relapse.

Answers to the question of "who takes care of whom" may be much easier to find for the person who is addicted but does not have a mental illness. Tough love has long been touted as the way to help addicts "find their bottom." Even in cases such as this, however, a family may find it difficult to know the point at which the addict's judgment is too impaired for the individual to be able to make proper decisions about caring for himself or herself.

How much more difficult are these issues, then, for families of dually diagnosed people? How can a family use tough love on someone who is actively using cocaine and also delusional? Families often want to believe that their family members can control their addiction even if they cannot manage their mental illness all of the time.

It is important for people with mental illness and addiction as well as their families to remember that both addiction and mental illness are diseases. Most important, they are diseases that need to be treated together, not separately. Unfortunately, in many states today, these treatments are not always offered together. Too often, addicted mentally ill people find themselves in a confrontive addiction group that may cause them to feel unsafe, and thus drop the group. Often, even in twelve-step meetings, mentally ill addicts may feel they do not fit in, particularly if they are not completely stable on their medications.

During the time I treated dually diagnosed people in an inpatient setting, I witnessed many heartbreaking scenarios. I saw mothers who were unable to retain custody of their children because of continued psychiatric hospitalizations. Once out of the hospital, however, these same mothers risked losing their children again because they would resume using drugs. The stressors of motherhood, financial problems, and the social stigma faced by someone who "cannot get it together" all combine eventually to cause such mothers to lose their children for good.

Caught in such a scenario, a mother may feel she has no real reason to "get straight." She may very well have come from a dysfunctional family herself in which one or both parents were addicts or mentally ill. Having children may have represented, to her, the first time she felt loved and in control of her life. Losing these children (and being told it is her fault) can often cancel any hope she holds for the future.

Another scenario that I have witnessed is the individual who enters treatment so that he or she may return to live with the family. The family, however, burned out after years of struggling to assist the individual in maintaining stability, may not allow the person back in the family home, no matter how well he or she does in treatment. Family members may be convinced that, if the individual had stayed away from drugs (or alcohol), none of this would have happened; thus, they may conclude that it is no longer their role to provide support for something the person brought on himself or herself.

Although it is true that the abuse of drugs and alcohol is not conducive to stability in someone who is mentally ill, addiction is not usually the cause of the mental illness. However, sometimes individuals who are mentally ill and addicted may continue to use drugs or alcohol within the structure of their families so that they may appear more "normal" to those with whom they live. This drug use may or may not be in conjunction with taking prescribed psychotropic medications. Individuals may repeat treatment episodes time and time again with the primary desire to remain in the family home. In the family home, however, their behaviors, even when they are sober and stable on medication, may still prove frustrating to their families, and, therefore, they may retain the sense that nothing they do is enough.

Another common scenario is when husbands or wives come into treatment and openly admit that they are there because their spouses said they would leave them if they did not get help. Unfortunately, summoning up the motivation to do the hard work of recovery can be difficult when everything depends on whether someone else will stay or leave. Some of my patients struggled to get well and maintained months, even years, of sobriety and stability and still their mates left. Sometimes, too, when people become sober and stable they may realize the relationships they set out to save are unhealthy, and they become the ones to end the relationships. Although people may seem to enter treatment for all the wrong reasons, many times the end result can still be health. As a counselor, I try not to judge a person's motive for getting treatment.

What is the answer, then, to our initial question about caretaking? As much as possible, I have tried to teach the people with whom I work that their most important and true home is inside themselves. People in the throes of active addiction often become spiritually bankrupt; they no longer have any sense of self-worth, and they become accustomed to searching outside themselves for meaning. In our twelve-step program, we teach that individuals who are members of Alcoholics Anonymous (AA) or Narcotics Anonymous (NA) are willing to become family to those seeking to address their addiction. Sponsors (people who have been sober and offer to guide others through sobriety) can be mentors and family as well. A home group (meetings held on a weekly basis) can be a touchstone for people who want to know themselves and measure their progress. Most important, twelve-step programs teach that one must come in contact with a higher power to help the individual as he or she tries to achieve quality of life.

I do not mean to imply here that people should merely pray to rid themselves of mental illness and addiction. What I do mean is that building a support system outside the family of origin is essential if people are to be successful in recovery. People who are not in recovery from addiction often have difficulty understanding the rigors of staying sober.

I often encounter people with mental illness and addiction who do not feel comfortable in traditional AA or NA meetings. Common today are twelve-step programs with meeting attendees who may have to be on psychotropic medications and this is not viewed as compromising their sobriety. Still, those who suffer from paranoia, severe mood swings, or delusions are generally uncomfortable in the twelve-step group environment. In our New Jersey treatment program we hold Double Trouble meetings that cater specifically to people who are dually diagnosed.

Specific mental illness support groups can be accessed online through New Jersey's (or any other state's) Self Help Group Clearinghouse. Some examples in New Jersey are GROW (for prevention and recovery from depression, anxiety, and other mental health problems), the Depressive and Manic Depressive Association (DMDA), the Depression/Anxiety Support Group, Choices (support for depression), Parents of Bi-Polar Children, and many others. Unfortunately, it is often difficult for dually diagnosed people to address addiction issues comprehensively within these groups because they may not have the opportunity of working with twelve-step sponsors who are dually diagnosed even though they have a good understanding of mental health issues.

WHO TAKES CARE OF WHOM?

As much as possible, individuals with mental illness and addiction need to find ways to care for themselves, perhaps better than ever before in their lives. They need to find faith that a higher power is there for them, whether that be the group, a sponsor, or their notion of God.

What, then, is the role of the family? Just as we teach dually diagnosed people the need for acceptance of themselves and their illness if they are to achieve full recovery, families, too, must learn to accept these people as they are, people with whom they may or may not choose to live. They may do this through attending groups such as Al-Anon or the National Alliance for the Mentally Ill (NAMI). They may do this with the help of their church or a counselor. Certainly, they may choose not to do this at all. One basic truth, however, is that most people, if they are to have quality of life, need to experience love and acceptance from important people in their lives. Families who become educated about the mental illness of a family member as well as about the dynamics of addiction stand a better chance of accepting the recovering dually diagnosed person than the families who choose to remain in the dark.

Guilt and shame often can be deterrents to change for dually diagnosed individuals and their families. Parents are often afraid they may have done something to cause their child's illness. They may fear that, somehow, they are not doing the right things to help their child get or stay well. These beliefs may translate into self-consciousness about their child's behaviors and lack of acceptance of the possibility of relapses, regardless of how hard everyone works.

Rather than focusing on who is to blame for what, families and individuals with mental illness and addiction would do best to build their own separate support systems and then work to accept one another as they are. Dually diagnosed individuals should learn to admit how some of their behaviors can be frustrating for their families. They could even choose, finally, to live separately from their families so that they can enjoy short periods of quality time with their families when they are doing well. Group homes, halfway houses, and many other kinds of supervised-living situations often are the answer to this quandary.

Once the family and the dually diagnosed individual become educated about the nature of the disease of addiction and the person's specific mental illness, they may begin accepting what some reasonable goals for living might be. Maybe the individual will be able to work part- or full-time, and maybe not. Maybe the person will be able to remain out of the hospital for long periods of time, even for good, and maybe not. If both the dually diagnosed person and the family can decide to focus on the progress the individual is able to make in conjunction with his or her capabilities and limitations, frustrations may begin to diminish. It is important for the family to know what progress means for this person and to acknowledge it. It is important for the person who is dually diagnosed to do his or her best to try to move forward and be compliant with treatment, by working with a support system consisting of twelve-step meetings and a sponsor; doctors, counselors, and perhaps an outpatient program; and a supervised-living situation.

Such support systems have, as a common goal, the regular acknowledgment of an individual's strengths, encouraging the person to take part actively in decisions concerning his or her life. These support systems and the family can assist the dually diagnosed person by providing empowerment. Individuals who manage their own lives to the fullest extent are able to begin to feel that they have substance after all, and that all the powerlessness they have felt can be managed through seeking daily support.

In the vignette that follows, you will meet Beverly, whose story exemplifies the difficulties families and dually diagnosed individuals experience when asking, "Who takes care of whom?" Beverly's experience depicts the cycle of guilt, shame, and punishment that can exist from generation to generation when the need for acceptance and empowerment of the individual is not recognized.

Beverly's Story

The last time I remember seeing Beverly was during her fourth stay in our MICA unit. An African-American woman in her midforties, Beverly was the mother of three grown children, one of whom housed and cared for Beverly when Beverly was not smoking crack. Primarily, Beverly had a habit of coming into our rehab facility to satisfy her eldest daughter whenever she, once again, told Beverly that she would have to clean up her act if she did not want to be homeless. Beverly had been diagnosed with paranoid schizophrenia in her early twenties. She was unable to remember the number of psychiatric hospitalizations she'd had, but she did know that some of them had been for as long as eighteen months, an unusual length of time in this day of deinstitutionalization. Beverly's baseline (or usual mode of functioning), even at her best, was not good. Even when Beverly was compliant on her medication and not using drugs, she was paranoid, constantly heard voices, and had difficulty remaining in touch with reality.

Over the years I had become familiar with Beverly's story in a hit-or-miss fashion. She'd been assigned to my caseload each time, so I'd gradually been able to build some trust with her and to get a sense of what her life had been and was like.

Although Beverly's difficulty with trust was clearly due to her schizophrenia, I could not help but feel that the traumas she had experienced as a child were also a big part of her illness. Beverly's own mother had been diagnosed with schizophrenia shortly after Beverly's birth. Beverly, when she would talk about it, remembered a toddlerhood rife with warnings and suspicion. Beverly and her two younger brothers spent days at a time locked with their mother in her small, cluttered apartment. Drawn shades and furniture shoved against the door were always present in Beverly's memories. She told me those memories were a strong trigger for her to smoke crack.

I was reminded of how many of my patients tried so hard to re-create their childhood because it was familiar. Abuse can be familiar and sometimes even, in an odd way, reassuring. As a child grows, systems of reward and/or punishment occur and reoccur and finally become entrenched. The child comes to expect abuse if it is a pattern over a long enough period of time. Abuse can provide a kind of closure for a person who is accustomed to it and may have grown up feeling he or she deserved it. Later in life, the abused person may even gravitate to a significant other who will repeat the familiar abuse pattern.

Beverly had grown up afraid and cautious. She'd been in and out of foster homes because of her mother's hospitalizations. Neither she nor her two siblings had any idea who their father was. They never knew when their mother might come out of the hospital and reclaim them for a time, only to wind up being reimmersed in her world of horrors.

Beverly had her first baby at the age of fifteen. She named the child Angela because the child had seemed like an angel to her, someone who would love Beverly as she had not experienced love before.

As with so many of my clients, Beverly was more willing to get clean and sober for someone else than she was for herself. Maybe that's why her longest clean time after each of her previous stays had been no longer than six months.

I'd hoped that Beverly, as an inpatient, would find support in the on-site Double Trouble meetings we held twice weekly. It was clear, observing her in her first meeting, that being surrounded by a roomful of people she did not know was frightening for her. Halfway through the meeting, she asked me if she could go to her room.

Later, she admitted that going to any kind of twelve-step meeting was very difficult for her. As part of her outpatient program she had attended numerous meetings in the past, and Beverly confided that she always felt as if she did not belong there. She explained that she often felt the people were looking at her or talking about her, and she threatened to leave the outpatient program if she was forced to go to meetings.

For Beverly to learn about twelve-step principles and build a support system, I believed that she would most likely need constant repetition of what to do and what not to do in order to stay sober. Further, she would need small groups of people who knew her well and whom she trusted to be there for her.

In one of our dialogues I asked Beverly why she smoked crack when it clearly angered Angela and also made Beverly more paranoid. Beverly spoke of the sadness that would come over her which only crack seemed to take away. She told of how her children treated her as if she were the child— not letting her have any money; talking about her when she was in the room; accusing her of using crack when she was not. She spoke of how angry they got when she would finally resort to prostitution to get money for herself.

I was hearing the same self-defeating story I had heard with so many other addicts, particularly the most disenfranchised. Prostitution often became as much of an addiction as the drug habit. It was a way to make quick money and, sometimes, a way, no matter how unsatisfactory or rudimentary, of connecting. Beverly, who had the concrete mode of thinking that sometimes comes with schizophrenia, lacked the insight to see how this kind of behavior might be wrong or hurtful to anyone but herself.

Beverly explained that smoking crack was the only thing that would make the voices go away. Upon probing, I was able to get her to admit that, more than anything, she wanted to lift herself up out of the doldrums she experienced when she thought about her life.

During the times when Beverly was able to talk to me, she spoke of what it was like for her during those early years when her children were small. She had not been diagnosed with her illness until her children were seven, five, and three. The children's fathers had been in and out of Beverly's life only briefly and she had worked very hard to earn money and take care of her kids. She told of how she'd clean houses and take the smallest children with her during the day. She admitted that, when she had to work at night, she would sometimes leave the children alone in the apartment, but she always locked the door.

As Beverly spoke of how she had held down a job and cared for her children, I could see the pride and joy in her face. It was clear that she very much wanted to be that person again—someone who could make a contribution.

Beverly added that she had not used drugs when the children were small. She admitted that the crack, alcohol abuse, and prostitution had begun after the onset of her illness. When Beverly had to be hospitalized, and her kids were taken away, she was reminded of the hard years spent with her own mother—something she'd sworn she would never go through again.

Recalling memories, Beverly began to appear sad, and I knew it was time to change the subject. When I asked if she had pictures of her grandchildren to show me, she brightened and led the way to her room. Taped to the wall near her bed was a flurry of smiling faces, young and old. We stood awhile in silence as I admired her family.

I reflected, standing there, on how I knew this woman but did not really know her at all. This affectionate Beverly, proud of her family, wanting to get well, was not the Beverly who might, within hours, be paranoid, guarded, and craving to use crack. I knew how to be present only with her there and to listen.

Before Beverly could complete this last course of treatment, she had to be transferred from our rehab to our mental health unit. She became too unstable for us to manage her and, once again, we lost touch. Perhaps I will see Beverly again in a few months, or perhaps I will read her obituary. I will remember, however, all those smiling faces taped to her wall as evidence that this "crack mom" was a real live woman who loved and was loved.

Though Beverly is a constructed example, I encountered at least a dozen Beverlys during the time I provided inpatient treatment. I witnessed repeatedly the generational nature of the effects of dual diagnosis. What happens in a family when patterns of dysfunctionality are repeated generationally? I knew of Beverly's childhood, but what about her mother's childhood, and her grandmother's? It was clear from Beverly's story that her children and grandchildren represented her hope. Perhaps that had once been the case for Beverly's mother when she gave birth to Beverly.

Continuing the pattern, just as Beverly never learned to accept her mother's illness, so, too, had Angela been unable to accept Beverly's. She saw Beverly's behavior as acting out, treated Beverly as a child, and took primarily a punitive approach, perhaps believing she was exercising tough love. It is easy to see how these negative behavior patterns become further entrenched in a family when the message being communicated is that it is the family's job to take care of the dually diagnosed person. Families may be uninterested in finding out about alternative living situations because of their long-held guilt and sense of obligation.

In Beverly's case, Angela was likely continually frustrated by all the hope Beverly had placed in her from her babyhood on. Her attempts to fulfill that hope were manifested in letting Beverly return to her home again and again. The family was on a treadmill, going nowhere but afraid to get off.

With close supervision and careful case management, Beverly might have a chance to find out what her strengths are. Living separately and experiencing day-to-day successes as reinforcement, Beverly might begin to see that she does have the ability to nurture and love herself, with help. This would not mean that Angela, Beverly's other children, and her grandchildren could no longer be a part of her life. On the contrary, as Beverly becomes more independent and happier with herself, she might even begin to be a parent and grandparent in the truest sense of the words—something she had always discussed wanting to do.

Families and people in recovery may need to put aside old notions of obligation and duty and explore new ways of finding balance in their relationships with one another. Halfway houses, group homes, supervised-living situations of all types are available to dually diagnosed individuals in all states. It is imperative that families research these places and consult doctors and therapists about their appropriateness for their family members. Also, it is important for a change in thinking to occur on the part of the recovering people and the families. The truest way of loving someone is letting that person realize his or her own potential.

I do not mean to imply that dually diagnosed people must always separate from their families to get well. But dual diagnosis, as we have seen, affects the whole family system. Every person in the system must begin to examine the appropriateness of old ways of thinking and acting so that quality of life may begin to evolve for all.

Despite the devastating nature of these diseases, it is possible for recovering individuals and their families, if they exercise respect and civility toward one another, to find balance and actualization in their lives.

Kahlil Gibran, in *The Prophet,* expresses this most eloquently:

> But let there be spaces in your togetherness
> And let the winds of the heavens dance between you.
> Love one another, but make not a bond of love:
> Let it rather be a moving sea between the shores of your souls.
> Fill each other's cup but drink not from one cup.
> Give one another of your bread but eat not from the same loaf.
> Sing and dance together and be joyous, but let each one of you
>   be alone,
> Even as the strings of a lute are alone though they quiver with
>   the same music.

WHEN IS TOO MUCH HELP NO HELP?

In answering this question, I would like to stress the importance of the dually diagnosed individual's need to reconnect with others as he or she recovers. Reconnecting happens more readily as the individual becomes able to achieve a sense of self and accomplishment. When families and/or support systems continue to do things for dually diagnosed individuals when they can function for themselves, it may be difficult for the recovery process to be initiated, much less for it to progress. Families who have witnessed continuing relapses into active addiction and recurring episodes of active mental illness can understandably have difficulty believing these individuals have the survival skills needed to continue to change in positive ways.

Over time, family members may begin to invest large parts of their own identities in caring for the dually diagnosed individual. What begins as an honest fear for the individual's well-being may evolve into behaviors that family members incorporate into their day-to-day lives, sometimes without awareness of the negative effects of these behaviors on the dually diagnosed person, who may assume a dependent role that invites caretaking by family members. Ultimately, family members may begin to feel uncomfortable or angry as the person experiences prolonged periods during which he or she is able to function on a higher level and to make independent decisions.

What could explain this type of response from caring family members? Don't we all want to see people we love get well? To understand this phenomenon, it is necessary to explore how family systems operate. In family systems therapy, it is common to compare the family system to a wind chime: When a breeze blows and moves the wind chime, all the components produce varying sounds that together resemble music; sometimes a stiff wind may cause the sounds to seem more similar to noise. In any case, the wind activates all parts of the wind chime because they are connected, and, therefore, a system.

Just as each part of the wind chime has its own tone according to how it is constructed, so, too, do individual members of a family automatically take on roles when particular events occur. Members of the family may not discuss or even recognize their roles but, over time, in many families, the roles become firmly established and family members' reactions predictable when certain situations arise.

Another family systems concept is that of the "hero." This is the person in the family to whom everyone turns when a crisis arises. Conversely, another person in the family may be the one who gets into trouble often or is frequently unable to cope. If the recovering individual becomes this designated person, the whole family system will be required to change when the person becomes substance free and stable on medication. Family members who have been accustomed to scapegoating the person who is dually diagnosed may resent or be confused by the recovering person's new, more positive role in the family.

This can be frustrating and angering to the dually diagnosed person, who is working hard to become stable and independent. People with mental illness and addiction are often accustomed to hearing expressions of disapproval and disbelief:

> "You never stay sober more than ninety days!"
> "Did you forget your medicine again? You're acting strange."
> "You can't even keep your room at home clean. How do you expect to maintain an apartment?"
> "Do you really expect me to believe you're going to AA meetings every time you go out?"

For someone in early sobriety, comments such as these can reinforce long-held feelings of shame and inadequacy. This is the primary reason why the mentally ill addict needs to have a support system consisting of people who understand dual diagnosis, either because they are going through the illnesses themselves or are trained in the field.

This is not to say that families do not need a support system as well. It requires a giant leap of faith for families to adapt to new roles in a system that may have appeared to operate smoothly for years. It also takes patience and hope for family members to struggle (and sometimes flounder) in the process of achieving wellness and independence. It seems so much easier (and perhaps even more caring) just to step in and closely monitor the recovering individuals' medications, drive them to doctor's appointments, and make major decisions for them.

In many ways, family members can become dependent on a recovering person's remaining needy and/or ill. A parent who has spent years caretaking an adolescent or adult child may be accustomed to this child's company, the structure and meaning that caring for this child provides to their life together, and the excitement or familiarity of ongoing crisis. Family members may become accustomed to disability income from the recovering person and the individual may feel this pay is something owed to the family as part of his or her assumed role in the family.

The vignette that follows presents Jesús's story, which exemplifies some of the points just made. Jesús lives with his mother and he encounters, in treatment, an unresolved conflict inside himself that does not allow him to make the changes that would promote wellness for him.

Jesús's Story

Jesús came to our program directly from jail, and he would not be free to move back into society until he had finished a twenty-one-day rehab program. This was not Jesús's first jail stay. I saw, reading his records, that he'd been in jail off and on practically every year for the past ten years. Thirty-five years old, he carried a diagnosis of schizoaffective disorder. This disorder can be, for some people, a fairly severe mental illness similar to schizophrenia.

Sometimes Jesús would be profoundly depressed. At other times he would be hyperactive and unable to rest or sleep. It was often difficult for Jesús to distinguish between what was real or not real, and, frequently, he believed people were trying to hurt him. Sometimes he heard voices or saw things that were not there.

When the time came for me to meet with Jesús for his first counseling session, I could not believe this was the guy I'd been reading about. Neatly dressed and carefully groomed, he sat across from me waiting politely for the questions to begin. His brown eyes were alert and communicated warmth to me, even though he could not meet my gaze for any length of time.

He told me that he was actually grateful to be in rehab as he had not been doing well in jail. He'd grown tired of having to "watch his back" and admitted that this had made his paranoia (which he reported having often) much worse.

Tentatively, I began to discuss with Jesús the crime for which he had been sent to jail. He had been jailed, according to the record, for assaulting his mother and sisters. It was hard for me to believe that the man sitting before me and showing me so much respect could have done such a thing.

I recalled, fleetingly, Jesús's admission late the day before. His mother had accompanied him onto the unit, and I remembered having been surprised and somewhat put off by the fact that she had presented the charge nurse with a large shoebox of various medications. She had firmly told the nurse to make sure that Jesús took the medications at the right times of day, pointing to a list accompanying the box. She had included herbal supplements, vitamins, and other potions she said he needed in order to function. She'd emphasized more than once that he would not remember his medications on his own.

As we had discussed the incident with Jesús's mother in a treatment team meeting, we had wondered if Jesús would have difficulty with our daily medication dispensation regimen, which required the patient to show responsibility for his compliance. From the first day, however, Jesús had shown up in the medication line along with the other patients, apparently willing to follow the same routine as everyone else on the unit. He'd been content with our explanation that his medication regimen while an inpatient would be limited to medications prescribed by our psychiatrist.

During our discussion of Jesús's assault on his family, he haltingly explained that he sometimes experienced these episodes of rage that caused him to lash out and hurt people—even those he loved. He admitted it usually happened when he was drinking.

I explored with Jesús his recent history of sobriety. He told me that three months was usually the longest he could go at one time. When I questioned what stressors he might be encountering at home, he briefly explained that he lived with his mom and sisters and that they were everything to him. He could not meet my eyes when he spoke of his shame over hurting them. He told me he felt he owed his family a lot for sticking by him and emphasized that he knew he'd never be able to make it without them.

Later in the week, I spoke by phone to Jesús's outpatient program counselor, who revealed that Jesús had grown up with an abusive alcoholic father who had beaten Jesús's mother on a regular basis. Jesús, the oldest of six kids, had felt responsible for her and had done all he could to protect his mother and provide for her.

Jesús had been able to hold jobs now and then for moving companies, and even after he began showing mental illness symptoms at twenty-two, he still kept going to work, trying to keep the family together. By the time he was twenty-five, however, the mental illness, with its accompanying paranoia, and all those years of suppressing his rage took their toll. Jesús's behavior had become more and more erratic, even though he had promised his mother after his father's death that he would always take care of the family.

Drinking became a way in which Jesús could calm the inner voices that destroyed his peace, but when drinking, Jesús would find himself repeating his father's hated behaviors—lashing out and becoming abusive. Jesús spoke to me of how he had sworn he'd never act the same as his dad. Yet now, more and more, he saw himself, despite his best intentions, drinking more and spending time in jails and hospitals. His mother had once told him that he had the same "devil" in him as his father. Jesús told me he believed it, too.

In our discussions, Jesús spent little time discussing the long periods during which he had been able to work and to stay compliant on his medications. He emphasized more how everyone in the family believed he was "disabled" and feared that, if he worked too many hours in a year, his Social Security disability check would be cut off.

As Jesús and I built trust during the ensuing sessions, we were able to tackle some discussions about what Jesús would want for himself in sobriety. He spoke of having a family, a place of his own, and a job. Momentarily, his face glowed, but then he quickly added that he did not know how he could cope with his anger without drinking. He did not appear to comprehend that all of the trouble he had gotten into had come after he drank, not before.

This anger Jesús spoke about was certainly not visible to us on the inpatient unit, as Jesús quickly made friends and created a three-week home for himself. He was elected community chairperson by his peers, people vied to sit at his table during lunch, and he was sought after by many female residents, who were captivated by his sultry good looks.

In one of our sessions, Jesús and I discussed relapse triggers. He admitted that having beer in the house was one of his strongest triggers. He said that his mother and sisters kept it in the house and that they did not think they needed to get rid of it just because of him. He spoke of how his sisters had pointed out that his outpatient program was supposed to teach him how to say no to beer.

I asked him what his mother thought about getting rid of the beer, and he shared that his mother did not want his sisters to get angry and leave. Jesús, his two sisters, and their three children lived in the house and paid for rent and food from their checks. They had promised Jesús's mother that they would take care of her in this way. Jesús emphasized that he felt that complying with his mother's wishes was the least he could do in view of all he'd put her through. He expressed disappointment with himself that he could not stay away from the beer when it was in the refrigerator and vowed that he would try to learn to be stronger while in this facility.

I had thought that Jesús was ready to discuss the negative effects of alcohol on him—how it was the source of a major part of the aggravation he caused his mother. But as I got to know Jesús better, it became clear that the real issue was how trapped he felt in a situation where he was unable to remain well. He told me how often his outpatient program counselor had urged him to find a place of his own and to return to work, but that he had been hesitant to renege on the promise he'd made to his mother, pointing out that his check was not enough to pay for a place of his own and to care for his mother. He also admitted that he needed the safety net of his mother and sisters; he believed he never would be able to make it on his own.

Jesús had reached the point at which he no longer wanted to try being out on his own, yet being at home was increasingly stressful for him in his role as the family "bad guy." It was clear to me and to everyone in our unit that Jesús was far from a "bad guy" when he was compliant on his medication, sober, and in a low-stress environment. I wished he could see himself as we saw him.

Close to the end of Jesús's stay in our rehab program, we were in a small group that was discussing whether liquor should be kept in the home of a recovering person. Jesús brought up the beer that was in his mother's house and the group loudly declared that it should be removed. They argued with Jesús that his family needed to know that he should not be tempted by beer in the house. Jesús became restless and I could see traces of the anger he'd described to me beginning to erupt as he felt himself being cornered by the group.

He launched into an outburst that was completely unexpected, accusing the group of trying to say bad things about his family. He told them they were just like the people in his outpatient program, against which his family repeatedly warned him. He said his mother had made him stop going to the outpatient program because they kept encouraging him to move away from home.

The group tried to probe Jesús's anger, but he shut down and would say nothing more during the session. After group, Jesús apologized to me for his outburst, but he said he would rather not discuss his living situation in treatment anymore. He thanked me for all he had learned in our sessions, but I could see the defeat in his eyes.

In another week Jesús would be through with the program. I felt there was little more I could do. Jesús was having trouble choosing between what his mother wanted and what he wanted for himself. The angrier he got about the life he'd been forbidden to have, the more he felt he owed his family, to make up for that anger. But when he drank, which he would probably continue to do, the anger came out as rage—rage that might ultimately take someone's life.

Certainly, it was taking Jesús's life. As I watched him walk down the hall toward the nurses' station, I thought of the connections Jesús had made in life. In spite of the very serious mental illness he had, he had managed to work, to make friends, and to remain out of the psychiatric hospital for long stretches of time. The most important connection of all, the one we all make with our families of origin, however, had stunted him. Maybe someday he would turn from it and seize his own life, but, I realized with sadness, it would not be this time.

Although it is difficult to understand wholly the point of view of Jesús's mother and sisters, their fear and frustration in the face of Jesús's continuing relapses and rage is understandable. As we seek ways to establish harmony in the family system, it is important to stress that we do not look for a place to put blame. The relationship Jesús has with his mother and sisters provides reinforcement for him and for them in many ways. Fear of change, failure, loneliness, or criticism from others may be keeping this family system frozen in place.

Because of the progressive nature of addiction, Jesús's life losses will increase if he continues drinking. Consequences such as jail, probation, and hospitalization will likely become more frequent over time. These worsening consequences will probably make inroads in Jesús's self-esteem and on his ability to manage his mental illness. If this inability (or unwillingness) to change continues, neither Jesús nor his family will see the new vistas that could lay ahead for them as individuals who are separate, actualized, and productive human beings.

For the scenario to change, Jesús's family will have to gain trust in the support systems available to them. From their report, Jesús's aftercare program had often reached out to Jesús's mother and sisters, urging them to support him as he sought independence. Consistently, this was received as interference. Jesús was told by his family that his aftercare program was bad for him and that he just needed to work harder to learn to say no to beer.

When families become entrenched in what is familiar, even when that is frightening and potentially life-threatening, their resistance to change may reach the point at which no support system can assist or intervene. Teaching families how to trust in one another and in support systems that can foster change and growth remains a major task for those working with people who are dually diagnosed.

WHAT HAPPENS WHEN FAMILY SEEMS TO BE THE ENEMY?

So far, in the discussion of the treatment of individuals who are dually diagnosed, I have emphasized the need for the individual to begin connecting (or reconnecting) with others to build the spiritual and emotional resources necessary for him or her to enter and maintain recovery. This process ideally is initiated in a person's family of origin as he or she grows and matures. However, an individual who is dually diagnosed often comes from a family in which mental illness and addiction (sometimes untreated) have been present—in parents, siblings, grandparents, aunts and uncles, etc. Much speculation surrounds the effects on individuals who grow up in households in which one or both parents may frequently be emotionally absent because of active mental illness or addiction. Children who grow up in such an atmosphere, with one or both parents unable to tend consistently to their emotional needs, undoubtably are affected in some negative ways.

How a child will react to a parent's illness often depends on that child's own emotional makeup. Some children learn to become caretakers. Others learn to act out in order to get attention. Some will adopt their parents' dysfunctional methods of coping, despite the pain they have personally felt as a result of these negative behaviors. I have had clients who reported having been introduced to cocaine, marijuana, or heroin by a parent, and others who have reported that their parents procured drugs and paid for their children's drug use so they wouldn't turn to crime. I have also had clients whose parents sexually abused them (or sold them to be sexually abused), with the payoff being drugs, money, or attention. What do these children learn? How can a system that requires trust to create wellness ever engage such children?

Can a dually diagnosed person's family actually appear to be the enemy? Perhaps the real enemy is the disease itself—whether addiction or mental illness or both—which causes generations of individuals to act and react dysfunctionally, to learn mistrust, and, ultimately, to feel hopeless about their own lives and the future.

Family members who are ill and/or have been abused themselves often have not learned proper ways of parenting or nurturing. Their children, in turn, often carry on this generational "curse." This does not mean that they have no desire for wellness, for change, or for hope. However, they often have little knowledge of how to begin to trust, connect, and escape the family's bondage to disease.

In the next vignette, you will meet Penny, a child of the kind of family system just described. Penny represents the apparent strength and determination of many children who come from a long history of abuse. On the surface, it is difficult to detect the hopelessness that is ever present in Penny. Easily activated and persistent, this hopelessness motivates much of her behavior. Plagued by a nagging sense of low self-worth, Penny helps others readily, appears to be a leader, and always has her defenses in place. In the end, though, for Penny, hopelessness wins.

Can this change? How can it change? What does an individual do without family members to help, when one's family actually appears to be a threat? What does someone do whose primary learned defense is offense? What can turn around the tendency to set oneself up for failure because the individual does not believe in any other way of being? As a treatment provider, I ask that question daily and wonder whether the only answer is, as heard in AA and NA meetings, "Don't leave until the miracle happens."

Penny's Story

When Penny entered our rehab program, her house was in foreclosure, she and her husband had declared bankruptcy, and the Department of Youth and Family Services had taken custody of her five children. The only way she was able to receive care in our unit was because she was one of the lucky few chosen to meet our charity care quota.

Penny told me in no uncertain terms the day I first met her that no one was doing her a favor. What she really wanted was to die. She spoke of how her husband had called 911 after her overdose on heroin five days before. Then he had left the home. The rescue squad had come and revived Penny and she has not heard from her husband since. She had been placed in inpatient treatment with little hope that anything was going to change. Dying was still very much on her mind, and she emphasized this to me repeatedly.

During Penny's eight-year marriage to Richard, running away was just one of the things he did to annoy her. Although Penny and Richard lived in a deceptively safe-appearing suburban area of New Jersey, Richard had dealt heroin, cocaine, and marijuana out of their home since they'd first been together. Until Penny, at nineteen, knew she was pregnant with their first child, she'd been one of his best customers.

She'd been determined to get through the pregnancy clean and sober and had achieved that. However, by her second pregnancy, she'd been diagnosed with bipolar disorder (a mental illness characterized by mood swings from depression to mania) and her doctor had recommended medications. However, being afraid that medications might harm the fetus, she had not taken them. She told me of the ups and downs of her moods while she had been pregnant and of the increasing tension between her and Richard, who just wanted her to be as docile as she had been when she'd used drugs with him.

Between pregnancies, Penny had tried mood stabilizers, but the responsibilities of her growing family and Richard's refusal to work and his troubles with the law made it nearly impossible for her to deal with the chaos in her life. Penny's doctors had told her that her medications could work better for her if she did not have so much stress. She told of how, when Richard would be in jail, she'd be on the phone trying to collect drug debts owed to Richard so she could use the money for his bail. In between, she said, she went to bake sales and PTA meetings and tried to figure out what to feed the kids and how not to lose the house.

During our sessions, Penny told me of how she'd been raised in foster homes because of her own parents' drug problems. She told me of years when she had lived briefly with her dad while her mother was in the state psychiatric hospital. He had shared a bed with her when she was five and six years old and had routinely sexually abused her, with penetration. She showed no emotion as she told me of this but did say that he was now in prison and she was constantly afraid he would look for her if he got out. She said that he had come by the house one time after she was married to Richard; he had been high on something and had approached her sexually. Alone in the house and pregnant with her third child, Penny had been forced to have sex with her father once again—this time oral.

Penny, who had been shuttled from one foster family to another in her younger years, had done poorly in school, and she reported that her moods had been "all over the place" during those years. By ninth grade, she had dropped out of school, was smoking marijuana daily, and was picking up whatever odd jobs she could. She told me that, during a period of cleaning houses, she'd gotten sent to juvenile detention because she could not help stealing things from the houses she cleaned.

Penny went on to tell me how much she'd planned to change once she had a chance to have a family of her own. She spoke of how she had not wanted to subject her children to what she had gone through in her childhood, but lately she was becoming more and more convinced that she'd probably just been fooling herself.

Back then, however, she'd given it a shot. Once out of juvenile detention, Penny had been placed in a work-study program where she began learning hairdressing. She said that her inability to read well and her tendency to fly off the handle had made learning tough, but she had persevered and finished the course.

Then Richard had come along to get a haircut one day, and Penny had been dazzled. Eight years older than Penny, Richard had done construction work with his dad on and off for years during high school and after. When his father had died suddenly of a heart attack two years after Richard graduated from high school, Richard's mom had moved to North Carolina to live with her daughter's family, turning the family home over to Richard.

Penny spoke of meeting this "together" guy who had had his own home at the age of twenty-five. She said that, after the first haircut she'd given him, Richard had kept coming back to the beauty school and asking for Penny. She'd thought that, finally, things were beginning to go right for her. She and Richard had started dating, and at first Penny hadn't thought too much about all the drug trafficking. Richard had continued doing construction jobs now and then. Then, however, they both had gotten deeply into heroin.

She told me that she'd known, two years into the marriage, that things were not right. She told of Richard's stopping working. He had even begun to bring other women into the house, she told me, her expression unreadable. He'd been disgusted by her moods, he told her. He would hit Penny and she would hit him back. She told me that the kids had seen and heard the fights, and that she had begun to see that she was harming them, despite her urge, since their conception, to protect them.

Penny spoke a lot in our sessions about her fear that she would never get her children back. She did not even know where they had been placed and had not seen them in weeks. She said that she had been too unstable for so long that her children's caseworker wouldn't arrange a visit. She wondered aloud if she would ever again be stable enough to be in her children's lives.

She spoke of how marijuana kept her calm and how she'd used it to cope with the stress in her life. Then she had gotten strung out on heroin, and the kids had been taken away, Richard had left, and now there was no home to return to. In Penny's mind, everything had ended, and she had little hope that she would be able to turn anything around.

Penny, however, was good at "faking it 'til you make it"—a popular twelve-step admonition. She took on a leadership role in her rehab program. Her feedback in group appeared honest and courageous, and her treatment of even her most annoying peers appeared fair and patient. Knowing what she had gone through in her life, I asked Penny if she had ever received therapy for the abuse she had experienced. She denied that she had and insisted that she never would. She was determined, she said, either to pull herself together or to die. Clearly, her ability to trust was presently too impaired for her to be able to avail herself of any long-term therapeutic intervention.

Penny's progress on the unit was short-lived. By the tenth day of her stay she was unable to sleep, hypertalkative, and irritable. She engaged in grandiose behaviors and seemed to be approaching a full-blown manic episode. When I spoke with our staff psychiatrist about Penny's mood change, he told me that some patients, such as Penny, "rapid cycle"—meaning that they can have several manic or depressive episodes within a year. He stated that Penny's life stressors, plus her hopelessness about the future, made it difficult for her to get and stay sober. Her recent heroin overdose, her long history of drug abuse, and her rundown physical condition did not help matters any.

In a manic state, Penny was not as easy to talk to, and I began to see that her appearance of "having it all together" had been a facade. She walked out of groups she found uninteresting, she paced the halls at night, and she was caught smoking. Usually our unit policy was to discharge someone immediately for smoking. Sometimes, when a person had absolutely no place to go and was willing to sign a behavioral contract, we gave them another chance. In Penny's case, I appealed to the treatment team to give her another chance.

Despite her severe and persistent mental illness, Penny's drug and legal problems had caused her to be turned down repeatedly for Supplemental Social Security Income. She had no income, was not well enough to work, was not eligible for psychiatric hospitalization, and had to be put on a waiting list for a Volunteers of America shelter. I thought, if I could just see her through treatment, I might be able to get her into a newly formed, free Christian treatment program. Little information was available about this program, but I'd been networking to find out if Penny could be a candidate for it. A careful reading of the program's goals and objectives gave me the impression that the program could provide Penny with much-needed stability, increased self-esteem, and an environment, a halfway house, where she could be rehabilitated over a period of months.

I told Penny about the program and we sent in an application so that we might do a telephone interview together with the facility to see if Penny could be eligible for admission. Even though the facility was in another state and Penny dreaded the thought of further losing contact with her kids, she was willing to give the facility a try.

To get into the facility, however, Penny would have to complete treatment and be stable on her medication. Penny signed a behavioral contract and, in the ensuing days, calmed down somewhat. She and I were both on pins and needles about the telephone interview because there just were not many other treatment options out there for Penny. She did not look good on paper and she had no income. I didn't have a clue that the one thing that would end up keeping her out of the facility was, ironically, her long list of medications.

Three days before Penny was due to be discharged, the facility we'd been trying to get her into decided, "after much consideration," that Penny was just too sick and too much of a risk for them even to interview. We called Penny down to the treatment team meeting that morning to discuss her options. In the three days we had left, we knew that it was unlikely we would find much more for Penny than a bed in a shelter and an appointment with the welfare office. Once again, she would be back out on the street, she would not have enough money to purchase her many medications, she would not have the emotional stability to get and keep a job, and, worst of all, she would be, again, completely alone.

Penny walked into the room that morning, trying hard to mimic her old jaunty saunter to show how cool she was. I could tell by the way she sat on the edge of her chair, grinning sarcastically, that she was going to act out. We'd only just begun to discuss her refusal by the program and her options when Penny stood, shook her hair out of her eyes, and delved deep into her jeans pocket. She told us that she wanted to make things easy for us. Withdrawing a rumpled pack of cigarettes and a lighter, she defiantly stuck a cigarette in her mouth and lit up. As she strode to the door she commanded us to throw her out.

Before anyone could stop her, she plowed her way down the hall, through the disbelieving patients scrambling to get out of her way. Great plumes of smoke followed her, a first on our unit, and Penny's statement of what she thought of us, the system, and, sadly, herself.

I stayed in her room while she packed. She gave me the cigarette and let me flush it down the toilet, but regardless of what I or anyone could say, I knew she was leaving our voluntary unit. Despite knowing what would make her well, Penny, and the system, lacked the resources.

A social worker from our unit agreed to drive Penny to the county offices where they could look into getting her some help. I knew, however, that, as she had just done, Penny would probably continue to sabotage herself. She hadn't had the time or wherewithal to help herself be healthy enough to learn other ways.

For someone with a persistent recurring mental illness and an addiction problem, a support group is integral. Throughout her life, Penny had tried, most of the time, to be her own support system. In so doing she had managed to develop some strengths, but her recurring illness and the pervasive hopelessness that plagued her from time to time kept her from realizing those strengths.

One of the biggest needs for clients such as Penny is a continuum of care that provides lengthy aftercare, regardless of ability to pay. Penny's long list of medications should have been a motivating factor for treatment to be provided. Sadly, the extent of her illness (and her manipulative and socially unacceptable behavior) kept her from receiving treatment. This is often the case for dually diagnosed clients, particularly those who are said to have "burned their bridges."

For Penny, acting out was a way of life. No one had ever taught her how to move forward in productive ways. She had been unable to sustain hope or make right choices for any length of time. Her lack of trust had kept her from bonding in her foster homes, in twelve-step programs, and even, to a large extent, on our unit. Penny's economic poverty and her illness might just condemn her to an ongoing poverty of spirit. If all men and women are created equal, how can this be so?

WHEN FAMILY MEMBERS DIE, THEN WHAT?

I often remember a story I heard early in my counseling experience that caught my attention. A counselor I worked with spoke of a patient of hers, a woman in her forties, who had finally "gotten her life together." For years, this woman had been in and out of psychiatric hospitals and detox centers and in legal difficulties. Now, suddenly, she'd managed over a year of sobriety, was holding down a responsible job, and appeared to be remaining stable on medication. Naturally, I wanted to know what magic the counselor had wrought to assist this woman. (Back in those days, I thought counselors could work magic; now, of course, I know better.) She told me, "It wasn't anything I did, and I don't even believe it was anything she did. The fact is, the patient's mother died, and she finally had to grow up!"

I have to admit that sounded pretty simplistic to me, and a bit coldhearted as well. Now, after years of counseling, I have come to find that the intricate ties among family members can impede wellness, foster it, or sometimes have little effect at all. Few of us think, when we are with our families, how our not being around would affect them. It may seem morbid to us to forecast what life for our husbands, children, or parents would be like if we were gone.

Families may think there will always be someone around to look after their members who suffer from mental illness and addiction. They may believe that siblings, cousins, or family friends would naturally want to take on this role, and perhaps they would. If, however, dually diagnosed people are automatically labeled as people who need looking after, they may be deprived of the chance to experience life to the fullest extent possible. How can they begin to know what their limitations and strengths are if they are not able to interface with the world around them as we all do?

Dually diagnosed individuals and their families should consider whether they may have become enmeshed in their relationships. Sometimes this insight can best be accomplished through family counseling that addresses everyone's needs and decisions they will make on how to fulfill them. Because family members may voice differing needs and goals, they will need to work on ways to "agree to disagree." Family members may have difficulty believing that the dually diagnosed individuals will be well enough to exercise good judgment in pursuing their goals and needs.

Within the dually diagnosed person's family, some members will have differing viewpoints about what should be done to ensure that the dually diagnosed individual remains safe. Information on dual diagnosis is available in community mental health centers and through specific support groups for various mental illnesses. Al-Anon and Nar-Anon provide education for family members about ways of helping people with addictions realize their strengths. It is essential that families and people who are dually diagnosed avail themselves of all the knowledge they can as they assess the health and wisdom of their interactions.

For dually diagnosed people, stress and change can be important factors in relapse. Since eliminating stress from anyone's life is unlikely, the most we can do is to empower people to deal with what occurs in the best way they can. Empowerment can come to dually diagnosed individuals from counselors, their families, and themselves. If a person does not want to explore or use his or her strengths, there is little chance of recovery. I have often heard counselors say, "The patient is just not ready to get well." How can we know, though, when years of conditioning within the family of origin may have convinced the person that he or she does not deserve wellness, is weak, is useless, has no willpower. What does it take for a patient to be ready to be well?

Throughout these pages, I stress the importance of empowerment for the person who is dually diagnosed; it may be the only "magic" a counselor can work—to be a part of this empowerment process. Twelve-step programs, regular psychiatric appointments, aftercare programs, community support systems, and mental health organizations (such as NAMI) must all be a part of the dually diagnosed person's repertoire as he or she seeks quality of life. In the case of the patient who became more able to cope after her mother's death, we will never know the exact dynamics that came into play, or even if the mother's death was a direct factor in the person's decision to pursue wellness.

Dually diagnosed people and their families must realize that, regardless of the seriousness of the addiction or the mental illness, these individuals still need to learn how to use every resource they have, every support system they can find, and every ounce of inner strength they can summon to be, in and of themselves, as well as possible. This is a daily fight. Although it is difficult to watch our children struggle, it is easier than sitting still and doing nothing. That kind of inactivity does not foster feelings of well-being, it is not actualizing, and it is not life-giving.

The term *life-giving* arises from my work with a particular type of inpatient. This patient was ready, even eager, to die, although not in poor health, in deep legal trouble, or without resources. Usually, such a patient had no clue about how to recognize the flickering ember of hope inside himself or herself and fan it into a blaze. In fact, often the patient could no longer see the ember or maybe was unaware that it ever existed at all. I've seen this response in twenty-year-olds, forty-year-olds, and I saw it in Eleanor, a patient of seventy-eight, whose story follows.

Eleanor's Story

The first time I saw Eleanor in the hall I had a fleeting thought that she might be a new staff member. But she couldn't be! She was at least seventy-five years old and looking pretty decrepit at that. By lunchtime that day I was informed that Eleanor was in rehab to get off a benzodiazepine (used for sedation) and that she would be part of my caseload.

Eleanor, who was actually seventy-eight years old, sat across from me looking as if she could not fathom what she was doing in such a place as our rehab program. For at least three hours, she reported bitterly, she'd been making her way up and down the halls amid crack addicts, schizophrenics who were talking out loud to their "voices," and tattooed young men with multiple body piercings. She told me in a low voice that she wanted to go home and that she could not understand why her children had put her in such a place. She quickly informed me that she was not interested in answering any of the intake questions I had for her, as she was certain a mistake had been made and she would soon be leaving.

I had to admit that I kind of agreed with Eleanor, but I wasn't going to let her know that. I tried to reassure her by promising that we would spend a lot of time together, that I could help her to relax and sort things out, and that she would have a chance to rest here and get away from her cares at home.

Eleanor did not agree. She argued that there was no way she was going to feel better if we insisted on taking her medicine away from her. After some questioning, I determined that by "medicine," she meant her benzodiazepine. She insisted that it was the only thing that would let her relax or sleep since her husband, Fred, died three years ago. She said that she could not understand why her children hated her taking the medicine and were demanding that she go to rehab to get off it.

I'd read Eleanor's chart and had seen that Eleanor's children, both in their forties, had become increasingly concerned about their mom over the past three years since their father had died. They reported that Eleanor had been using benzodiazepines around the clock, sleeping through the days and not answering her phone when they tried to reach her. She'd been falling and had received several minor injuries in the past year. Recently, she had even managed to finagle more than one doctor to prescribe benzodiazepines for her when her prescriptions ran out early—a ploy addicts are known to use.

When I mentioned these things to Eleanor, she was defensive. She told me she needed the medicine and that it did not matter anyway if she slept all day. She insisted that she had nothing left to live for now that Fred was gone. She said her kids had their own lives and a lot of her acquaintances were deceased. She firmly concluded that when she thought of how things used to be, she just did not want to go on.

I told Eleanor that benzodiazepines often made depression worse rather than addressing it. I emphasized that Eleanor had made herself so tired from all the benzodiazepines she'd been taking that she no longer had the energy to want to build a life of her own. I shared what her children had said to me about their desire that Eleanor learn how to make a new start and find out what life could hold for her without Fred.

Eleanor looked doubtful. Later in counseling, I would learn that Eleanor's dependence on Fred (and on her parents before Fred) had been so strong that she had never really known what a life of her own could be like. Eleanor's present problem with the benzodiazepines was a symptom of a deeper underlying problem that Eleanor and I would come to address in the weeks ahead.

If a person suddenly quits a benzodiazepine after depending on it for years, he or she can be at risk for a seizure. Because of Eleanor's age and her long use of the benzodiazepine, she had come to us from a three-day detox program where they had begun gradually weaning her off the benzodiazepine and had started her on an antidepressant. She showed little excitement when I shared that we would be keeping her on the nonaddictive antidepressant, even though she complained that she did not feel safe without the medicine to which she had become accustomed. I reassured her that we would keep her safe while making the switch from a medicine that had become an addiction to a medicine that could give her the energy and impetus to make a new life for herself.

Eleanor gave me her opinion of how safe the rehab facility looked to her. She doubted she could even sleep at night, she said, with all the "strange-looking" people walking around. She informed me that sleep had been a problem for her for a very long time, and that this was why she'd been increasing the benzodiazepine. She expressed doubt that she would be able to sleep at all without it. Following her transfer from the detox center, she reported sleeping four or five hours a night.

Even though a lessening need for sleep can be typical for someone Eleanor's age, an addicted person used to long periods of sedation often reports having feelings of deprivation and fear. Eleanor was experiencing the typical reaction to reduction of a benzodiazepine drug. Her body had become used to large amounts of the benzodiazepine, and now that we had reduced the amount she was given, she had begun to feel withdrawal symptoms, such as anxiety, tremulousness, sleeplessness, and depression. Our psychiatrist had expressed concern that we not attempt to withdraw Eleanor too rapidly, as it could be very hard on someone her age.

One of Eleanor's biggest problems was that she had become used to instant gratification. Whereas she had felt almost immediate sedation from her benzodiazepine, the antidepressant we gave her was not having anything near the same effect. She'd hoped for "instant happiness" and instead felt the energized, somewhat "hyper" response common in people when first taking antidepressants. That, combined with continuing withdrawal symptoms, was causing discomfort and confusion in Eleanor. She wanted to know *exactly* when she was going to start feeling better—a question I could not answer.

I finally did manage to build enough trust with Eleanor so that she was able to commit to stay on the new medication and remain on the unit. It was clear to me, however, that this was a half-hearted commitment. She still hoped she could talk her kids into taking her home and letting her resume her life as it had been. I could see we were going to have a lot of work to do together.

As the days passed and Eleanor got to know the staff and patients, I was encouraged to see how she slowly began to brighten. Always accustomed to arising early, she was one of the first patients in line in the mornings for her medication and the nurse's monitoring of her vital signs. For the first time in a long time, Eleanor had a reason to get dressed in the mornings. She arrived at breakfast, gray curls shining, her freshly pressed house-dress immaculate. Her peers were amazed. They gave her compliments she'd probably never heard before, such as, "You are one cool chick" or "Look how good you got it together!"

Eleanor quietly thanked them for the compliments, smiling shyly. From my vantage point in the cafeteria or in the halls, I often speculated whether this type of social interaction was mostly new to her. Could it be that, at seventy-eight, she was having some of her first meaningful interactions with people who were around her on a regular basis?

When I asked her this in our next counseling session, Eleanor told me she had always been shy and "moody" in school and that her family had protected her. She had dropped out of school in tenth grade, had never had many friends, and had met Fred through her father, who had employed Fred in his accounting firm. She told me that she'd gone straight from her parents' home to living with Fred and that he had, in many ways, taken over protecting her.

Eleanor confided that her family had always known, and Fred had seemed to know, that her moods, her shyness, and her nervousness made things harder for her than for other people. When she'd had each of her two babies, her mother had come to stay with Eleanor and Fred for several weeks each time. Eleanor said that many of the child-rearing responsibilities had been taken over by Fred, who'd opened his own accounting practice in their home.

When the kids had had problems, they had gone to Fred. When Eleanor had had problems she, too, had gone to Fred. In a later session, Eleanor finally confided that Fred had "somehow" gotten her the benzodiazepines and that she'd been dependent on them long before his death. She told me that he had called them "nerve pills," and she admitted that she'd been taking them for ten years before Fred died. She said that he had liked her calmer and that she, too, had felt better about herself on the pills.

As Eleanor talked, I envisioned what her life must have been like. A mood disorder that was probably a treatable illness had somehow caused her to be labeled as "less than," someone who had little to contribute. Little wonder she needed her pills to feel better.

In rehab, after venting some of the things she had to me, Eleanor became even more interactive, telling me she liked the way it felt to be with other people on a regular basis and to have something to offer. She brought pencils to group, something no one else seemed to remember. In the evenings, she sometimes helped some of her peers do their homework from the workbook our rehab program provides. In a small-group session, in the second week, Eleanor shared her story with six of her peers, relating how she had depended on her pills more and more and that she knew now she had become addicted to them.

Her peers said that whoever had prescribed the pills to her was just like a dealer. After thinking about that for a while, Eleanor said that she wondered now what the past thirteen years of her life might have been like without the pills. She admitted that she had been scared to try anything new, scared to commit to anything, and unable to see herself as having anything at all to contribute.

Her peers were amazed, each one volunteering a way Eleanor had helped them since she had been in rehab with them. She had truly earned a position of respect during her two weeks on the unit, and she was experiencing, clean and sober, the unique sense of self that had been so long lost to her. Eleanor admitted to the group that she needed to be at this rehab. She said the pills were only a small part of what was wrong with her. She did not go into detail, but she knew I was aware of what she meant.

As more time passed, Eleanor stopped being so guarded. She opened up about how much she had underestimated herself all of her life. When they visited, her children noticed the difference in her and commented on it. Watching Eleanor talk animatedly with her grown children, I realized that they, too, had been cheated by rarely, if ever, having experienced the superb mothering, comforting abilities, and good judgment that I'd watched Eleanor lavish on her younger peers in rehab for the past few weeks.

By the time Eleanor's three weeks in rehab were over, we had her off the benzodiazepines and beginning to acclimate on her antidepressant. She was sleeping through the night, her gait was steady, and she appeared to have a better understanding of why the benzodiazepines had not been helping her. She knew now that they had been meant to tide her over during those few difficult weeks after losing Fred. Her doctor had not known that, over ten years, Eleanor had already become dependent on her "nerve pills." She realized now that she had lost valuable time out of her life because of them.

We were able to get Eleanor into an adult aftercare program following discharge. She would be transported daily to a place where she could be with people her own age. They would monitor her antidepressant and address any other health-related needs she might have. She would be stimulated daily to remain connected with others.

On the day Eleanor left, she came to my office to say good-bye. She thanked me for helping her see that she had abilities, worth, and something to offer. Watching her walk away, her posture confident and her stride energetic, I thought of how important it is for a person to have the gift of self-confidence. For Eleanor, it was a gift that almost came too late.

It may be true that Eleanor is different in some ways from the dually diagnosed person who experiences persistent recurring symptoms and/or is cross addicted to more than one substance. Who can really say, however, how impaired or intact any of us are when we have not been nurtured to be ourselves? Eleanor brought to her relationships with her husband and children a limited sense of her own self-worth and of her ability to make a difference. Placing blame on someone for how or why this happened is not important. For Eleanor, however, as with the woman whose story began this chapter, it took someone dying for her to identify and embrace her own desire to live.

Chapter 2

Reasons for Resisting Treatment

"If you had a terminal disease and someone came up with a medication you could take to be well, would you take it?" Many lectures that I gave on our inpatient unit began with this quote. Of course, patients were always quick to point out that the question was silly and irrelevant. Who *wouldn't* take a medication to save his or her life?

However, when I would go on to point out that addiction is a disease and the tools that treat addiction (twelve-step meetings, sponsors, abstinence, etc.) are the medication, patients were also quick to roll their eyes, become distracted, or tune me out. The dually diagnosed client also faces the issues of the mental illness and the need for medication and ongoing therapeutic support. For individuals with dual diagnosis who had endured trial after trial of psychotropic medications, multitudes of styles of case management, and myriad life losses, the thought of there being a "cure" of any kind that would have long-lasting results was often one they had abandoned years before they came to me.

Why would people give up hope in their ability to be well? Most addiction treatment providers agree that the desire for control is a primary factor in why an addict uses. For dually diagnosed individuals, who may come from families with a history of mental illness and/or addiction, feeling out of control of what was going to happen to them was a daily reality. Looking for a way to feel secure or even to not care so much, many individuals who have grown up with unpredictability and lack of nurturance will search for ways to numb their feelings. If, then, addictive tendencies do develop, it is because using the substance (or the process) becomes, for a time at least, a means of discovering or predicting what their feelings will be. Thus, dually diagnosed individuals may experience frustration in recovery when told, "What you really need to do is *surrender*." For people who have spent much of their lives longing for some control and who have become accustomed to finding a quick but false sense of security from substance abuse or dependency, the rigors of twelve-step recovery often seem unreasonable and perhaps even impossible.

Despite the vow children may make early on not to be drunks, as their parents were, sometimes offspring in families in which addiction is present do find that drinking or using drugs (ironically) seems to provide a quick and easy answer to the emptiness one feels from not having had emotionally present parents. Children of addicts often become addicted themselves, learning that this is a short-term way to have at least some predictability in their lives. They can predict how they will feel and are better able to buffer themselves from the sharp edges of reality that have been prodding them for many years. Thus, addiction may begin. If later diagnosed with a mental illness, addiction may serve for a time as a tool for inducing sleep, managing mood swings, avoiding life consequences, and, finally, assuaging those "not okay" feelings people can have when they are continually told they are different.

Dually diagnosed individuals need courage and trust to put aside their methods of coping, which they have used for years, even though they know these methods no longer work for them. Their defenses will tell them that all these methods still do work; that others do not have the answer, nor do they care; that the old easy ways of feeling good—whether that was sliding into oblivion or simply "getting high"—are still the best means of coping.

Even though individuals who are dually diagnosed know on one level that they need to abstain from mood-altering substances and comply with their medication regimen, they often do not realize, at first, the difficulties they will encounter. For example, they may not be able to summon the trust to work with a twelve-step sponsor and/or a psychiatrist who dispenses medication and urges the patient to tolerate side effects. Liquor is, indeed, quicker.

For families of dually diagnosed individuals, this inability to enter recovery and remain in recovery on the part of their family members is often frustrating and difficult to understand. "Why don't they just listen to the doctor? Why don't they just go to meetings and stay clean?" Family members, however, may not understand that starting a medication can, for many days, make people feel "not themselves." New medications can cause side effects that dually diagnosed individuals may feel unable to tolerate. A caring, available, and patient treatment team can assist patients through the regimen of adjusting to new medications, to sobriety, and even to "being present in real life" on a full-time basis. Patients may say that they want to be able to do these things, but they may also have a multitude of mixed feelings and fears when they enter the process.

Counselors encountering patient reactions to this process may say that the "patient is resistant to treatment." This phrase implies that the patient does not want to get well, or that he or she is not invested in doing the work. It may imply for some counselors that the person in treatment will be manipulative, untruthful, and generally uncooperative. This assumption is unfair to the patient and not conducive to success in treatment. Resistance to treatment is a natural part of the patient's defense process—the only means he or she has of "keeping it together."

To achieve success in addressing resistance to treatment, counselors must remember that they need to "meet the patients where they are." Empathy is key. As much as possible, counselors should get within their patients' reality, feel their fears, and, most of all, care about them. Patients recognize caring—or lack thereof. The counselors, doctors, and family members who will succeed in helping dually diagnosed individuals work through their treatment resistance are those who agree to be companions on the journey.

The following vignettes provide examples of what being a "companion on the journey" means. Dually diagnosed individuals face fear of change and loss of control, so their resistance to treatment—if tolerated, examined, and even, at times, embraced—may be an important key to success in treatment.

IF I GET WELL, WILL I LOSE CONTROL?

In facing resistance to treatment, we often do not conceive of the patient as being appealing, easy to like, and someone who ultimately will assist us in *preventing* him or her from getting well. Individuals such as Melanie, whose vignette follows, will sometimes go to great lengths in treatment to maintain their known survival techniques. For this patient, who had been abused in childhood, her way of staying "safe" was based on a carefully maintained way of rationalizing her behaviors and her lifestyle.

Because Melanie was bright, she managed to convince us, as she complied with every aspect of treatment, that she was actually willing to change and grow. In reality, Melanie wanted only for her addiction to be removed. She did not want to face the fear and vulnerability that her addiction covered. As is the case with many people with addictions who come into treatment, Melanie wanted something "magical" to occur so that she could stop using cocaine but not have to examine her life. Unfortunately, as is verified by twelve-step programs, stopping using is only a small part of recovery; the main part is willingness to change, a part Melanie could not and would not accept. For a brief moment during her stay with us, I sensed the magnitude of the inner turmoil she had kept secret, even from herself, and I wondered when, if ever, she would be able to face it.

Melanie's Story

I knew as soon as I met her that Melanie would be a joy to work with in treatment. She'd signed up on the board on my office door for an appointment as soon as she'd unpacked and gave every indication of being all business and ready to learn what we had to teach. As so often happens to me when I meet an overtly cooperative individual such as Melanie, all thoughts of the patient's having any resistance to treatment leave my mind. I would later recall that extreme cooperation can be one of the primary ways in which people maintain control in their lives.

Unlike many who come to our rehab program, Melanie had not opted for the "casual look." Dressed in a white blouse and a well-fitting navy skirt and matching vest, she resembled more an executive secretary on her way to work. I assessed her to be around thirty-five as I glanced at her well-made-up face. Her skin was smooth and unlined, her blonde hair neatly tied back in a low ponytail.

I began our interview by reviewing with Melanie the reasons why she wanted to get off cocaine. I asked her what form of cocaine she used and the frequency and amount. Melanie stressed that she freebased cocaine and her demeanor was somewhat haughty as she said this. She stressed that smoking crack was something she would never do. (I've found almost a class distinction among drug users concerning the kinds of drugs they use and how they use them.) She told me that she used nearly every day, spending at least $200 a day, or more if she had the money.

Mentally I calculated this at $1,400 per week—a pretty hefty salary for anyone. I commented that this must be a serious financial drain for her and asked if this was the main reason she wanted to quit. Melanie assured me that she made enough money to support a far bigger habit than that. Her main complaint was that the cocaine made her edgy and paranoid and that she could not afford to be that way in her line of work. She went on to tell me in a matter-of-fact way that she was a prostitute and that she was very good at what she did—when she was not paranoid from using cocaine.

It wasn't that I didn't meet prostitutes on a fairly regular basis among my clients, but they were usually downtrodden young women—often mothers of several kids—who'd been forced to sell their bodies to support their drug habit. Occasionally, I'd seen women who swore, no matter what, they'd never sell their bodies for drugs. Their next time back in rehab they'd admit with shame that they'd finally had to resort to prostitution. Here was Melanie, though, speaking calmly about her "profession" and how drugs were getting in the way.

Curious as to the forces that had propelled Melanie into such a life, I began to discuss childhood issues with her. She told me that her mother had raised Melanie alone. Her father had left the home while Melanie's mom was pregnant with her. Melanie said that she and her mother had lived with her Uncle Todd, who baby-sat Melanie while Melanie's mom worked at night as a waitress. She was quick to say that her mother had spent a lot of time with her during the day, and that she thought her childhood had been pretty normal. She said that her mother had married a few years back and now had two sons.

During the time when Melanie had spoken of her Uncle Todd baby-sitting her she gazed out the window behind me, a detached expression on her face. I wondered if she might be disassociating and asked for more details about how long her Uncle Todd had been a primary caretaker for her. She said he had been in her life from the time she was a baby until she was around six. She was clearly uncomfortable discussing this, and I filed that fact away in my mind as I moved on to a more comfortable topic.

We completed the interview with Melanie recounting her years in high school and the backseat she'd had to take with her mom after her stepfather and her two younger brothers came onto the scene. She'd gone to community college but had dropped out after meeting a man who'd introduced her to prostitution. She told me that this man was not a "pimp," but someone who had known she could make a lot of money and had steered her in this direction.

Following our initial interview, I thought about some of the hunches I'd had about Melanie while listening to her. Her tendency to disassociate at times while talking to me made me wonder if she'd had a history of abuse. This would explain the paranoia she spoke of when using cocaine. Checking through Melanie's records I saw that she'd been given a diagnosis of post-traumatic stress disorder (PTSD).

As I got to know Melanie better and she let her guard down, I began to notice a kind of fragility about her. For all her sophisticated knowledge about the world of prostitution, she was clearly vulnerable and hurting. I thought I'd begin addressing this vulnerability by focusing first on the cocaine, since that was her main concern. I asked Melanie how she had gotten started using cocaine. She told me that, as a prostitute, she was often invited to snort cocaine with her johns with the promise that it would make everything better. She said that snorting cocaine had removed her inhibitions at first so she got into the habit of it, later moving on to freebasing as her tolerance to the drug built. She went on to add that the cocaine didn't really make sex different for her, as she had always liked sex a lot for as long as she could remember.

When I asked Melanie when she had lost her virginity, she reddened and said that there was a lot she could not remember from her childhood and that, anyhow, she could not see the point of trying to remember. She said that, though she often wanted very badly to be touched and to feel close, she would find herself flinching away from her partner and she did not understand why this was so, except that she knew cocaine made her paranoid. She went on to insist that using cocaine was the only real problem that she had, and she did not understand why I was going so deeply into her childhood issues.

When I asked Melanie why she thought she had been given the diagnosis of PTSD, she gave me a flat stare, commenting that the doctors probably had to come up with some diagnosis to get her into rehab. Again, she urged me to talk just about the cocaine and how she could get off it. We spent the rest of the session talking about ways Melanie could recognize relapse triggers and exert refusal skills. Because she didn't intend to stop prostituting herself, she'd be exposed to cocaine on a regular basis, and she accepted this.

One afternoon I was showing my group a movie on bipolar disorder, *Call Me Anna,* the story of Patty Duke's childhood, which portrayed some of the childhood abuse she went through, including sexual abuse on the part of her foster father. I sat next to Melanie while the movie was showing, and I watched her as she drew her feet up underneath herself. She began trembling and finally covered her face. I could hear soft sobs coming from behind her fingers. I signaled to another counselor in the room that I was leaving, escorted Melanie from the room, and walked with her to my office.

We sat together for several moments while she cried and tried to stop shaking. She finally was able to ask me what I thought was the matter with her. I repeated the question back to her, and she talked a bit about the movie and how she'd felt watching Patty Duke as a small child suffering sexual abuse. She spoke about her mixed feelings of wanting to be touched and hating to be touched and expressed confusion about how she could have these two feelings at the same time. She looked up at me, her face contorted with tears. Finally she admitted to me that she felt her uncle had been the only person who had really cared about her. She spoke of how busy and distracted her mother had always been (and still was). She said that, when her uncle had touched her, she had felt as if everything would be okay, and that he had taught her things that she used as her means of earning a living now. She felt disloyal, she said, admitting these things to me.

We went on to discuss how she felt betrayed by her body now and that she did not understand why she flinched away from someone touching her. Even though we were able to establish that she had been frightened of being touched long before Melanie began using cocaine, she kept insisting that she knew, if she could get off the cocaine, she would be able to be "normal."

We began to talk about what Melanie saw as normal for her. She asked me if I thought a person could be a prostitute and normal. I was silent, seeing if she'd answer her own question. After a moment, she raised her head and looked at me. She told me tearfully that she had thought a lot lately of having a husband and kids but was sure that no one would want her now, after the life she had led. She added that she was used to the special treatment she got as a highly paid prostitute. She was used to the money and the attention. She said she did not want to give it up.

After a silence I asked Melanie how much of her real self she felt she gave to what she did. She thought about that for several moments and then answered that she knew her prostitution was like a mask she wore—not really her at all. She began to weep again, quietly this time. We sat together until it was time for the next group, and I noticed that her previously sleek hairdo had fallen into a messy tumble of curls around her face, her makeup had worn off, and her outfit was rumpled and askew. I felt that, with all we had said and with all Melanie had seemed to realize, we were beginning to make some progress. Maybe Melanie would be willing to explore underneath the mask with me. It seemed she was beginning to trust me enough to take that journey.

As so often happens when a patient sees so much so soon, however, Melanie retreated further than ever behind her mask of control. By the next day, she was pointedly avoiding me. She did not want to talk further about her uncle and she said in therapy group the next day that she thought that using cocaine was something she would probably have to accept as part of what she did as a prostitute. She told the group she did not need their feedback on this, and that she had decided to moderate her use and return to snorting cocaine instead of smoking it.

It was as if a heavy door had slammed. Melanie had glimpsed the child in her who had been flinching from the touch of men who were using her, as her uncle had. Desperately, she wanted to believe that the fantasy world she had created, where their touch meant admiration and even sometimes consolation, was real. She could not or would not let go of this now. Melanie discharged herself from our program by the end of that week. Her resistance to treatment had been that she was unable to let go of the safe-seeming world she had created for herself. Even though, in reality, this was not a safe world, it felt safer to Melanie than the alternative, which would have been having to acquaint herself with that trembling abused child inside, the one who flinched.

Had Melanie been a treatment failure? I did not think so. Melanie had seen what she could bear to see and she would remember. It was my hope and my prayer that others would come along (and soon) to encourage her in her journey.

For people who have known deep stress and pain, the journey to recovery often has to be made in increments. As a counselor I have often seen myself coming into a patient's life late in the journey, after much nurturing and care has already been given by someone else. I hoped that I had been someone who had treated Melanie gently enough so that she could continue to trust and eventually nurture the trembling child within her.

WILL I STOP FEELING NORMAL IF I STOP USING?

One of the strongest protests I hear from people entering recovery is, "I don't feel normal when I'm not using a mood-altering substance." Even when I ask clients to reflect on their earliest childhood years, they might say, "No, I never felt normal or okay inside myself until I began using drugs [alcohol]."

"Normal," to most of us, probably refers to the way we are used to feeling much of the time. It is, however, a relative term onto which people are likely to project their own meanings: calm instead of anxious, happy instead of sad, energized instead of lethargic. For a person who suffers from a chronic mental illness and an addiction, one thing is certain: Feeling "normal" is a key concern. The question "What does *normal* feel like to you?" should be asked and analyzed early in the treatment process for a person who is dually diagnosed.

In my role as a counselor I came to believe strongly that individuals who prioritize "feeling normal" are not just making excuses. They are truly terrified that they will not be able to stand the way they would feel sober and/or on psychotropic medications. For the person entering treatment, this fear is a major factor in what we call treatment resistance. Again, it should be remembered that treatment resistance, when correctly addressed, can provide insight into what the dually diagnosed individual is seeking in wellness.

Many issues come into play for dually diagnosed persons when discussing feelings. They may consider the feelings associated with their mental illness to be what is normal for them. For adults who have smoked marijuana daily since their teenage years, normal may be simply feeling slightly high every day. For those who have been depressed all their lives, the effects of an antidepressant may be felt as a relief or a threat. For people who have been addicted to heroin, normal means not being dope sick. For those with bipolar disorder, normal may mean looking forward to the bursts of energy and creativity common during a manic phase. Taking a mood stabilizer to even out their moods may cause them to feel flat and sluggish. These are only a few examples of what dually diagnosed people have reported to me when they consider the changes that may occur for them when they enter treatment. The operative word is *change*.

Just as people fear surrender, they also fear losing who they have known themselves to be. Ironically, this can be true even when they have suffered multiple life losses for being who they have always been. Normal, then, seems to be that to which we have become accustomed. It means knowing what to expect.

A primary tenet of twelve-step recovery programs is that one must begin to "accept life on life's terms." Each new day the person is to surrender to whatever may occur. The recovering individual admits powerlessness over the addiction and asks, each day, for help from his or her higher power in negotiating what life dishes out on that day. He or she asks for help in not using an addictive substance, regardless of the day's events. The next day is the same. For the person in a twelve-step recovery program, it is "one day at a time."

Learning to let go of control is an incremental process for many recovering individuals, as is being open to accepting unfamiliar feelings. This process may be far easier to accomplish when the dually diagnosed individual is in an inpatient setting and able to discuss side effects of medications daily with a counselor and a psychiatrist. If the patient is detoxing, he or she can discuss symptoms and learn about withdrawal and post–acute withdrawal on a daily basis. Most important, the patient will have continual reassurance that these withdrawal symptoms will abate if he or she stays sober and complies with the treatment regimen.

Increasingly, dually diagnosed individuals must seek treatment on an outpatient basis. They may return to work and go to outpatient groups at night for a few hours a week. Tolerating the side effects of new medications and staying sober when drugs and alcohol may be easily obtained is most difficult and requires careful case management. Dually diagnosed individuals can gain much as they discuss, in group therapy, the temptations and fears shared with their peers as they begin to accept life on life's terms. Dually diagnosed individuals in an outpatient program should work with a psychiatrist whom they can see on a regular basis and with whom they have built trust. Preferably, that psychiatrist will be affiliated with the outpatient program and will work with the addictions counselor providing group therapy.

As individuals come out of their addiction and become stable on a psychotropic medication, they may begin to realize that feeling normal, for most people, means being present to the daily roller coaster of life events and handling these events as they occur. For dually diagnosed individuals this may mean sometimes feeling overwhelmed, and having a support system will become an integral part of their lives. Having people to help them determine what medications to take, at what dosages, and for how long and to encourage them to comply with their treatment regimen will strengthen their ability to cope with life's occurrences. They will no longer need to buffer their feelings with a substance, a process, or a behavior to "make it all go away."

Not everyone chooses to give up this buffer. For those who do, much courage and tenacity is required. In the vignette that follows, I present the story of an individual who must learn to deal with anxiety, which is, for her, an intolerable not-normal feeling. Substance abuse and dependency became the only answer she could find, and she strongly resisted treatment as she was urged to consider other options to treat her anxiety.

Amanda's Story

Anybody who has ever had panic attacks can usually recognize when someone else is having one. The rapid breathing, the inward stare, the clenched hands, and the shaking are all clues to the inner turmoil a person is experiencing. Having had my share of panic attacks, I was able to recognize that the young girl sitting on the bench outside my office was in the midst of one. I sat down beside her and waited until she turned her head rigidly to look at me.

Quietly, I asked her if she was feeling scared. Sitting on the bench beside her, I could feel the quaking of her body. Her lips trembling, she told me that every time she tried to detox from alcohol she would feel worse and worse as the days passed. She said that she had been in a detoxification unit before coming to our rehab program and that they had told her she would be feeling better with each day she stayed clean and sober. Her eyes flashed with anger as she told me how sick she was of being told that she'd feel better without alcohol.

It was clear to me that her trust in treatment providers had been strongly compromised in the past few days. Wanting to rebuild that trust, I listened quietly, hoping she'd go on. She was lost in the throes of her panic, however, and she turned away from me and doubled over until her face was almost touching her knees. Loudly she moaned that she wanted to go home.

I asked for her name, wanting to personalize what I would say to her, and learned that her name was Amanda. I told her that what she really wanted, at the moment, was to drink and that if she left our unit feeling the way she did now, she would drink. I inquired whether she really wanted to lose the benefit of all the time she had already put into recovery.

She sat up and turned to me, her voice firmer now that her panic seemed to be abating. Loudly proclaiming that she did not intend to put up with feeling this badly for the rest of her life, she said that if drinking would make the panic go away, *yes,* she would drink. Angrily, she added that she was sick of everyone else thinking they knew how she felt or how she would feel with or without alcohol.

I was glad to see her anger. It was something I could work with. I told her my name and informed her that she was assigned to my caseload. I explained that, during her stay in our rehab program, I would to try to help her understand how she could begin to tolerate the way she was feeling.

Quickly, she asked if she could call her mother. Even though I could see from her demeanor that the panic had passed, I knew she wanted to make that one last attempt to duck treatment. I prayed silently that Amanda's mother would not rescue her.

While Amanda dialed her mom, I sat at my desk and glanced through her chart, which I'd gotten from the nurse's station. Nineteen years old and an honor student, Amanda had started her first year of college this past fall. She came from a family of high achievers. Her dad was an engineer, her mom a nurse practitioner, one brother was a lawyer, the other a stockbroker. Amanda, the baby of the family, had plans to become a pediatrician. So what was wrong with this picture? Nothing in the chart tipped me off to any family dysfunction except, of course, for the striving atmosphere that must have surrounded Amanda during her formative years. That, I knew, was only a supposition on my part.

I listened to Amanda's conversation with her mom as I read. She segued from demanding to be taken home to pleading. Silently cheering for Amanda's mom, I could hear, early on, that nothing she said was going to work. Amanda was with us for the duration. Finally, Amanda slammed down the phone. She sat slumped in her chair across from me, staring down at my desk, muttering that if she had anywhere to go she'd check herself out and take a bus. As she ran her hand through her short, curly hair, I could see that her nails were bitten to the quick.

I very rarely self-disclose in counseling—I'm aware that it is usually not advised, for good reasons—but I had an impulse now to share with Amanda. I told her that I understood how she had just been feeling as I had experienced panic attacks myself. She looked at me intently, some doubt on her face. I could see she wondered if I was bluffing in order to keep her in treatment. I went on to admit to her how, when I had felt that way in the past, I had been tempted to do almost anything to make the panic go away. Triumphantly, she said that then she guessed I also understood why she wanted to drink so badly. I told her I did understand it, but I also understood that drinking makes panic worse. She shook her head violently, saying that she should have known I would be just like all those other counselors in detox who had said that drinking was bad for panic. She insisted that, for her, it was different because drinking was the only thing that made her panic go away. She stood up, ready to leave, but I advised her to sit down a minute while I drew a picture for her. She became sarcastic, saying that a picture was just what she needed at the moment, but she did sink back into her chair.

I drew, on a piece of scrap paper, a series of peaks and valleys. Pointing to the peaks, I told Amanda that she was experiencing the rebound effect. The peak was her panic, I said. When she experienced it, she drank and came down to the valley (or temporary sedation from the panic). Then I added that, when the liquor wore off, she would peak again, only this time a bit higher than where she'd been at before. I pointed to a peak that was higher than the one before it. I explained to her that this was the way she built an increasingly higher tolerance to alcohol because over time she would need to drink more to get the same effect, and the peaks would continue to climb.

She stared at the paper, saying that she had thought her drinking had increased because she was older. I asked her how old she had been when she began drinking, and she admitted that she had been only nine. She said that she had been drinking every day for at least three years and that she had to drink in the mornings to stop the shaking and begin her day. As we spoke, I could see some doubt about the effectiveness of her drinking creeping in. She appeared to begin to see, gradually, that her daily drinking had become a job she had to do to function.

I asked her whether she had experienced the shakes in the morning since she'd left the detoxification unit, and she admitted that the morning shaking had stopped. That must be a relief to her, I pointed out, and she slowly admitted that it was. Having to admit what was good about *not* drinking was getting to her, I could see, and I decided that I wouldn't push my luck. Closing her chart, I told Amanda that we'd be meeting again later and that maybe she could think of more things that were good about not drinking.

She appeared faintly surprised that I was letting her off the hook so easily. As she stood to leave, she asked me whether the staff psychiatrist would be giving her something for her panic. I told her that antidepressants help sometimes and that certain antianxiety medications work for some people, but that her biggest need was to stop drinking and maintain sobriety. I encouraged her to talk to the doctor about medications. With a curt "Fine," she was out the door. As with many patients, she wanted a magic pill and she wanted it yesterday.

Throughout the rest of that day, Amanda stayed close to her room and did not mingle with her peers. It was clear she was in an almost constant state of panic, so before I left that afternoon, I went to her room to speak with her. She was lying on her side in a fetal position, her face buried in her pillow.

I told Amanda that staying alone worsened her panic, but she mumbled into her pillow that she just wanted me to go away. Ignoring her request, I asked her if she'd talked with our staff psychiatrist yet. She said he'd given her some pills that had not helped and she just needed a drink. Thanking her for her honesty, I emphasized that she did not *need* a drink; she just wanted one. She turned on her back, glaring up at me and loudly repeating that she knew when she needed a drink.

Appreciating the reappearance of her anger, I asked her what she had been thinking about before her last bout of panic began. She stared at the ceiling, then a tear trickled down the side of her face, and she told me that she was disappointed that the pill the doctor had given her did not work. She was remembering, she said, how nothing anybody ever gave her worked and she was afraid that nothing ever would. She was thinking, she added, crying in earnest now, that she would never be able to stop drinking because she could not stand the way she felt sober.

I agreed with her that those were panic-producing thoughts which probably would make most people feel badly. She turned her head and met my eyes, attentive now. I went on to propose another way of thinking. What if she decided to think that the medicine *would* work eventually? What if she chose to think that she *would* start to feel differently if she could commit to treatment here? What if she chose to believe that we might have some answers that she had not heard of before? What if she chose to think that she *would* be able to stop drinking if she listened to some of those answers we would be offering her?

She agreed that if she could have those thoughts, she probably would feel better. When I asked her casually if she was still feeling panic, she lay still a moment, staring at the ceiling, and then finally admitted that the panic was gone. Then, with a grimace, she said she could feel it coming back. When I asked her if she had allowed the old thoughts of failure to come back she nodded vigorously, excitedly verbalizing the insight that what she chose to think might actually affect how she would feel. She admitted that, for the first time, she was beginning to think that we might actually have some answers for her in this place.

I affirmed for her that, when she could begin to change her thoughts, she would go a long way toward conquering her panic. I added that, with therapy and medication, both of which we offered, we could begin to help her. She would have to be patient, however, because the effects would not be as immediate as those she'd become accustomed to experiencing with alcohol.

She'd turned on her side again, her back to me, but I knew she was listening. Telling her "good night," I left her room. Half an hour later, as I was leaving the unit, I saw Amanda, dressed and in the hall, shyly talking to one of her peers. At least she'd taken one piece of my advice. I hoped she'd be able to consider some of the other things she'd heard.

The next morning, Amanda was waiting in the hall outside my office when I got in. Huddled on the bench, her arms wrapped around her body and her hair uncombed, she looked as if she'd had a tough night. Unlocking my office door, I motioned for her to come in. As soon as she got into my office, Amanda said that the things I had told her were not working and that, no matter how hard she tried, she could not think about anything but how awful everything was. Sobbing, she told me she had not slept at all and that all she wanted was for her mom to come for her.

I knew from the records that Amanda's antianxiety medication, which she had been given for withdrawal, had been recently cut, and this would account for the increased sleeplessness and panic. I knew, too, that an SSRI (selective serotonin reuptake inhibitor) antidepressant might help her to begin to avoid the "awfulizing" she was doing, once it had had a chance to take effect. We talked quietly for a while, with me explaining how I could not call her mom at this time. I did offer to have her excused from some morning groups so she could get herself together and prepare to get to work. I said that what I needed in return was for her to commit to come in to talk to me every time she started to feel panic. I promised her that we would talk it through, as we had the day before.

Her eyes widened. Smiling shakily, she asked me if I knew what I was saying, because she'd probably be in my office all day long. It was maybe a weak attempt at a joke, but I felt a surge of hope for her success.

After Amanda had gone to breakfast, I went to a staff meeting where I recounted to the treatment team everything that was going on with her. The doctor prescribed a one-time nonaddictive sleep aid and an SSRI antidepressant. This kind of antidepressant is particularly helpful for people in early recovery in that it helps them to use the naturally occurring serotonin in their bodies in a more effective way. For a person in early recovery from addiction, whose serotonin production has been compromised over years of active abuse, the addition of an antidepressant with this effect can assist the person's recovery.

With the help of the sleep aid, Amanda slept most of the morning. By early afternoon, though, she'd been in and out of my office three times. Each time she felt the panic, she was overwhelmed by the same self-defeating thoughts—her belief that nothing we did for her would cause her to feel better and that she did not have much hope for herself. When I asked Amanda whether she thought she could begin to create hope with her thoughts, she smiled tentatively, saying that she was willing to try but that she was afraid of letting herself down.

For the next two weeks, Amanda and I met regularly at scheduled times and randomly when she felt the panic, episodes that began to decrease appreciably toward the end of the second week—something that Amanda noticed as well. She also noticed that she had begun to have more luck purposely turning her thoughts around when the panic began. I knew that maintaining sobriety and taking her medications was helping the therapy we were doing to succeed.

Amanda's parents came in, during the third week, to talk about her progress. Amanda's mom admitted that she had been nervous about coming to visit sooner for fear that Amanda would ask to be taken home again. Sitting across from her parents, Amanda had actually begun to look like the carefree nineteen-year-old she was. Her hair shone, her face looked relaxed, and the circles were gone from under her eyes. Amanda told her parents she was glad she had stayed in treatment and she apologized for all she had put them through. She said that she was finally beginning to believe that she could actually stay sober. Quietly, she admitted that she had not realized how much time and patience it would take, but that we had taught her how to think differently and how to "tough out" the hard times—which did eventually pass.

AA has lots of slogans for what happened for Amanda: "Fake it 'til you make it." "Bring the body and the mind will follow." Most of all, though, Amanda learned to connect with her own dormant belief in herself. This was one patient for whom I could report an excellent prognosis for recovery.

Amanda's story is but one small example of the struggle dually diagnosed people experience as they address getting clean and sober and stabilized on their medications. Someone as young as Amanda has, at least, the resiliency and the general good health of youth to help her along in this struggle. For multitudes of other dually diagnosed people who are older and have faced more life losses, including poor health, the struggle may be ongoing and difficult to resolve.

Family members of dually diagnosed persons can be most helpful by maintaining an awareness of how frightening this struggle can be. Not feeling normal may be a state of mind for which family members of dually diagnosed people have no frame of reference. Family members may believe that the terrifying nature of panic, mood swings, or ongoing voices in the person's head is something that the dually diagnosed person has caused through drug or alcohol use—"You made your bed, now lie in it!"

Dually diagnosed people and their families need to know that addiction is not usually the cause of mental illness. Certainly, addicts bring many of their life losses on themselves. Mental illness is usually worsened by addiction, but not necessarily caused by it. Sometimes mental illness may be masked by addiction, as the addict self-medicates symptoms for years. Often, once a dually diagnosed person stops self-medicating and begins working with a psychiatrist to find appropriation medications, he or she is more able to remain sober from mood-altering substances.

Medications, however, can have side effects, especially during the first few days of use. Dually diagnosed individuals need encouragement and someone to listen to their fears as they wait for side effects to abate or try out other medications. For people with a compromised sense of "being their old selves," reassurance and patience are key. Family members may believe that tough love involves telling someone to "get over it," but this approach is hardly effective when a person is terrified.

Dually diagnosed individuals who commit to treating their addiction and mental illness should understand that these frightening feelings will pass, and that time, the correct medication, and an understanding and patient support system can bring the promise of wellness.

WHO WILL I BE IF I GET WELL?

Treatment resistance can be strong for individuals who have used addiction, for much of their lives, to maintain a sense of who they are or want to be. For example, a young woman may form the pattern of using cocaine, methamphetamines, diet pills, or heroin to maintain her weight. After a period of time, the use of these substances may seem to be a necessary part of her daily existence. In this case, she becomes addicted not only to the substance but also to the results of the use of the substance, that is, weight loss. Another example is a shy, retiring young man who uses substances such as alcohol, marijuana, or cocaine to enable him to "fit in," or socialize, more effectively. He may find through using that he no longer has the concerns he had before about how others will see him. He can take more risks, speak up for himself more readily, and lose some of his inhibitions. For this individual, having to give up these substances because he has formed an addiction becomes a double loss. How will he now enter a room full of people he does not know and socialize with them?

Many young people today conceive of "partying" as using ecstasy at a rave, smoking marijuana behind the school or in a parked car, or attending an all-night keg party. How can young people successfully "party" without access to any of these behaviors? At eighteen years old it is difficult to comprehend that they are not the same as their peers, who will someday be able to put these substances down and move on with their lives. Young people who become addicted and find themselves facing the need for recovery experience many conflicting thoughts and feelings as they contemplate abstinence.

Some individuals are given mood-altering substances such as alcohol practically from babyhood. There may be virtually no get-togethers or transactions within their family structure that do not involve alcohol. People in this situation who become addicted to alcohol face the immediate problem, upon entering recovery, of how they will tolerate being around alcohol continually when they can no longer drink. They may have to contemplate not seeing their families regularly during early sobriety.

Individuals raised in painful childhood situations may have learned, early on, to self-medicate their emotional pain by using a substance. A woman may find that the use of this substance blunts the pain for her for many years until, one day, she finds she has become addicted to this substance and must give it up. She may very likely have had little opportunity throughout her life to develop alternate ways of coping with pain or trauma because of her habit of substance abuse. If, for instance, she began this sort of self-medicating at around the age of thirteen, she may enter recovery in her forties and be alarmed to find that she has little sense of how to deal with emotional pain or trauma in her life.

Individuals who are dually diagnosed, then, face not only this double loss of substance and lifestyle but also—sometimes for the very first time—being told they have a mental illness. For such people, even more than for addicts who do not have a mental illness, stopping substance abuse becomes an essential part of achieving good health. They learn that abusing substances will make the mental illness worse or that it will interfere with the effectiveness of prescribed psychotropic medications. They become informed about the physical, spiritual, and emotional losses that they may have sustained as a result of substance abuse, losses that compound when abuse continues.

Imagine the resistance such individuals feel when they enter treatment and realize that they can no longer look, act, or feel as they have in the past. Even if in the midst of sustaining considerable life losses because of their addiction, they may not know how to change—and they may not want to try.

Treatment resistance can be compared with the process of grieving. The person comes into treatment because of a loss and is angry, hurt, and in denial of that loss. More than anything, in the beginning, the person just wishes the loss had not occurred. It is essential that the treatment provider for the dually diagnosed person understand this response. It is important that families of dually diagnosed individuals understand that grief and loss are a process that takes time to complete.

It is unrealistic to expect the dually diagnosed person who enters treatment to stop using a substance (which may have in many ways defined that person) to be happy or grateful about being in treatment. The first question such an individual will usually ask is, "What can you give me that will work just as fast and just as well?" Unfortunately, this person may not be in the mood to learn how to postpone gratification, compromise, or substitute other behaviors or substances. Again, treatment providers and families of dually diagnosed persons must be companions on this long and often complex journey toward wellness—a journey that requires time, patience, and compassion.

The following vignette presents Candy's story. Candy developed a need for thinness due to self-esteem problems brought on early in her life. Being thin and attractive was, in the beginning, a way for Candy to get positive attention. She did not consider herself to be intelligent, having dropped out of school in the ninth grade after years of struggling. When she began focusing on looking good, being a good dancer, and attracting the opposite sex, Candy created an identity, finally, that pleased her. Fearing that she would gain weight if she gave up her addiction to diet pills, she resisted change, even when she found herself becoming psychotic.

Candy's Story

At only nineteen years old, Candy just missed being admitted into an adolescent rehab program. She came to us after months of hanging out at raves, doing ecstasy, "special K," and, worst of all, over-the-counter weight loss "medications." Candy was a dancer and she had come to our rehab program because she'd had a frightening psychotic break that had kept her in the state psychiatric hospital for the past two months. Now, in order to be released back to home from the state hospital, she would have to complete twenty-one days in rehab.

I'd seen Candy the year before when she had come to our program for just a few days and had signed herself out against medical advice. That time, Candy "had it together." Her luxuriant waist-length hair had been shining and always in place, her compact little body had been displayed daily in outfits that barely fit within our dress code, and her demeanor had been cool and superior. She made it clear, then, that she didn't belong with "these people."

During that stay she had been quick to tell me that she could make several hundred dollars a night as a dancer and that she was losing money sitting in the "nuthouse." So she'd checked herself out and had spent the last year of her life learning powerlessness.

She sat before me at our intake this time, and it was difficult to believe that this was the same person I'd seen only a few months before. Her hair was tangled and hanging in her eyes, her jeans were stiff with dirt, and her blouse was stained and baggy—but her eyes were the worst. Unfocused, seeming to stare inward, they did not connect with mine in any way. She seemed "not there," and I was unsure how to reach her.

I began by asking her why she had come back to rehab. I had to wait several seconds for her reply. Unable to meet my eyes, she said in a low voice that she had to be in rehab to get out of the state hospital, but that, honestly, she was afraid to leave the state hospital or even continue living feeling the way she did. I asked her if she had been clean and sober during the two months she'd been in the state hospital. (I knew she would have been able to get pills there if she wanted to.) She said she had been clean and sober but, even so, was still continuing to hear voices and was feeling frightened much of the time. She told me the worst thing, though, was that the medication she was being given in the hospital was making her fat.

Candy, at about five feet, six inches, looked to me as if she could weigh little over 100 pounds. I remembered her obsession with weight from the last time she had been with us. She had been found vomiting up most of her meals, that is, when she would even eat at all. I told Candy that she would need her medication in order to get well—that this would be a part of her treatment plan while in rehab. Looking at her chart, I noted that she had been prescribed a mood stabilizer for bipolar disorder.

Her voice rising, Candy said that when she weighed what she should and could look good and dance again, that would be when she could consider herself well. Beginning to sob, she added that everything was falling apart and all she could think about was dying. I believed her. Before she had gone into the state hospital, Candy had had a nearly fatal overdose. Then, her first week in the hospital, Candy had slashed her wrists, deep cuts that still were not completely healed. Candy continued weeping, softly asking why we wouldn't just let her die. She asked if she could leave my office, as there really was no reason for us to talk. I moved around next to her and sat in silence awhile, my hand resting on her heaving shoulders. Her pain was almost palpable, and I knew there was nothing I could say, at least not then.

It was difficult to get Candy to participate in the program in the days that followed. Clearly, she was hoping we would just discharge her back to the psychiatric hospital. In her mind, she had no clear future. I scheduled short, supportive sessions with Candy and didn't probe too much. I knew that her ego strength was low at that time and that she wouldn't be capable of much more than just making it from one day to the next. In the interim, I read her chart carefully.

Candy's mom had committed suicide when Candy was only five. Prior to that, her mother had been diagnosed with depression and alcoholism and had been hospitalized twice. During the hospitalizations and after her mother's death, Candy had gone to live with her father's mom, a woman who had consistently belittled Candy's mother and who had wound up raising Candy. A quote in Candy's file explained what it had been like for her: "She always told me I wasn't going to be useless like my mom. I had to be a good girl, get good grades, and look just right." Candy had done her best apparently but, from the first, she'd had learning disabilities and had been placed in special classes where she did barely average work. She'd dropped out in the ninth grade.

During our second week together, I began speaking to Candy about her childhood. She admitted that had been an awful time for her. She had missed her father terribly and could not understand why he would not include her in the new family he'd formed after her mother's death. She had described how young and attractive her stepmother was, stressing that her father had "eyes only for my stepmother." Her voice faltering, Candy told me she guessed that he had left her out of his new family because she was fat and dumb.

Candy continued, explaining that as she had entered puberty, everything began to change. She started to slim down and her beauty emerged. She found that, with some careful dieting and attention to herself, she could attract and interest boys and men. They wanted to date her and buy her gifts, and it seemed they were offering her a way out of the trap her life had become. She began to hope she would soon find a way to escape her controlling, disapproving grandmother.

She smiled as she told me she had never realized before how angry she had been with her grandmother for most of her life. She had felt great joy when she was finally able to detach from her grandmother and take charge of her own life—after she had found a boyfriend who took her to live with him and showered her with the first consistent attention and love she'd ever known. One way he had demonstrated his "love" for her, she said somewhat sarcastically, had been to introduce her to heroin and cocaine. Suddenly she had found her attention turned from her new boyfriend to her savior—a natural weight loss plan. Slimmed down, energized, and introduced to the "right" people by her boyfriend, Candy had gotten into the bar scene and had started dancing (her boyfriend had helped her to get a fake ID). She had begun to make a lot of money, which, of course, she had used to support both of their drug habits.

At first, she'd thought her life was perfect. She had a boyfriend at home who was attentive (when he wasn't *too* high) and admiring men longing for her as she danced. It had been, for a very short time, like a dream come true. However, soon she'd begun having trouble getting to sleep at night and had found that several nights would go by with almost no sleep. She had begun to get circles under her eyes that she could no longer cover with makeup and she had found that she was edgy and needing to be busy all the time. She said that she'd gone to a doctor who had sent her to a psychiatrist and that was how all her problems had begun. She'd been given medication that had "ruined everything," she said, because she immediately began to put on weight, to lose her energy, and, worst of all, she was told she was mentally ill.

She stared down at her hands, fighting back the tears. She had reached "perfection," she said, only to lose it after a few short months. When I reminded her that it was her grandmother who had introduced her to the need for perfection, she looked startled. She admitted that her grandmother did have something to do with her need to feel perfect. She stated that it had been an impossible goal—that she had never been able, in any way, to satisfy her grandmother. Underneath Candy, the dancer, she said, was no one at all.

Candy was spiritually bankrupt and probably had been for most, if not all, of her life. Spiritual bankruptcy comes when a person knows how to reach only outside himself or herself for satisfaction and identity. Seeking "things" and "relationships" and "processes" that have no real meaning, the person withers inside. The spirit lacks nourishment and the person's sense of self-worth declines. Further, as the person abuses substances and compromises his or her intrinsic value system, sense of self declines even further. Candy was accurately describing the way she felt. If she had not been an inpatient at that time, she probably would have turned quickly to substance abuse in order to feel better—and the cycle of inner destruction would continue.

As we proceeded in our counseling sessions, Candy revealed to me that, sober or not, on medication or not, she regularly took over-the-counter (OTC) weight loss pills containing ephedra. She also stated that, no matter what, she didn't intend to stop those pills: "I can't give up everything." In one session, I brought her a sheaf of papers from research about ephedra I'd done on the Internet. I spent time carefully explaining to her what the weight loss pills could do to someone with her history.

Candy wondered if this could be the reason why, even sober, she was experiencing anxiety and "voices." I told her that being on the OTC diet pills was not true sobriety. Candy's terrified expression told me that she had already begun to think about the weight she would gain and the control over her life that she would lose if she had to give up the pills. Quietly, I reassured her that with her youth and her history there was no reason she could not learn to control her weight in healthy ways.

More than that, though, I tried to help Candy address her inner self. Daily we talked about things Candy could remember from when she was a child, experiences that she had enjoyed and times when she had believed in herself. It was amazing to see how childlike she became during those talks, and I realized that, at that moment, she was that small, neglected child once again. With time and many sessions, I saw the little girl begin to grow up and become more sure of herself.

Toward the end of her treatment, I began to see a real change in Candy. She spoke with our nutritionist about a diet and exercise plan. She spent time with our psychiatrist discussing side effects and dosages of her mood stabilizer. Her grooming improved; she began to resemble more the nineteen-year-old she was and less the lost soul she had been.

Candy returned, at the end of her three-week period, to the psychiatric hospital. Together, we had discussed an aftercare program that would help her pursue her plans for recovery. The only thing remaining was for her to gain admittance to a halfway house for women. During Candy's stay, we'd gotten her on a couple of waiting lists but I knew, from experience, that halfway houses are cautious about accepting clients on medication—an all-too-familiar roadblock in treating dually diagnosed individuals. Candy planned to wait in the psychiatric hospital for admittance into a halfway house. She did not want to return to live with her grandmother and she had no job skills that would enable her to support herself.

I wish I could tell you that Candy is well today and has her GED (general equivalency diploma). I wish I could tell you that she has a good job and a nurturing boyfriend. As the case is with hundreds of dually diagnosed individuals I treat, I don't usually know how a client fares until, unfortunately, I see them back in our unit six months or a year later. Still, I do know that the seed I planted has at least germinated. I have no control over the kind of soil it will find. I just pray that Candy will be strong enough to help that seed take root and grow in her life.

Questioning one's identity is not something that is confined to people who are mentally ill and/or addicted. Our very sense of who we are is sacred to us and our defenses are always on guard as we attempt to create or maintain this often fragile sense of identity.

It is difficult to know how it feels to be someone who has sustained life losses or perhaps hurt someone as a result of actions performed in an alcoholic blackout or in the aftermath of a psychotic break. Who was the person then? How can the person make amends? Is change possible? Is medication the answer? For many dually diagnosed individuals struggling with a fragile sense of identity, treatment episodes that require them to self-disclose to near strangers and take medications that will change how they feel and behave are not only stressful but impossible to bear. A person who feels this way must be given options. Such a person needs to feel that he or she has choices and that those choices matter to and are respected by others. Learning to care about oneself and nurture oneself is a key part of recovery for the dually diagnosed individual.

In the case of Candy, self-nurturing represented just feeling okay about herself for the moment. In the short time we knew each other, she became aware that self-nurturing is really being there for oneself on a day-to-day basis, facing up to challenges, and postponing gratification. Being oneself is a long-range—lifetime—proposition that is filled with risks. Understandably, the person who at first resists treatment is afraid of those risks. Who would not be?

WHOM CAN I TRUST?

Individuals who are dually diagnosed resist treatment mainly due to their difficulty with trust. I've often thought that this difficulty with trusting people is not surprising, as addicted people may have consistently broken their own trust in themselves throughout their addiction. Further, they have probably violated the trust of those most close to them numerous times and no longer are sure what anyone may think of them. They may not even be sure what their own behavior will be in the future because their addiction has ruled them for so long.

In the behavioral health field, addicts are known for their tendency to be manipulative and dishonest. However, much of this behavior is a reaction to the way addicts think they may be seen and/or judged by others, even people who are trained to help them. Addicts often must resort to dishonesty and manipulative behavior to maintain their addiction, but this does not necessarily mean that they are inherently dishonest and manipulative people. Maintaining an addiction, over time, requires secrecy and negative life changes that often are contrary to the actual nature of the addicted person. However, addiction creates certain needs: the need to hide their increasing tolerance to the substance, the need for money to procure it, and the need, perhaps, to perform illegal acts to maintain a lifestyle that began as a choice and became an obsession. For addicts, then, mistrust is something that they are used to receiving from others, and as they continue in a lifestyle of which they may become increasingly ashamed, they begin mistrusting others and unable to let anyone know the depths of their despair.

Problems with trust are compounded for the dually diagnosed person. Medications used to treat mental illness can have troublesome side effects that may cause the individual to feel worse rather than better when the medication is first administered. Later, as medications begin to work, and the symptoms of mental illness disappear, the individual who has been accustomed to experiencing them may actually feel empty and alone. Individuals who enter inpatient treatment may experience fears of being taken from a safe place to unknown territory, where others act strangely. Withdrawal symptoms cause them to crave the security of home, or, at the very least, the opportunity to rest in bed instead of being required to attend groups that emphasize their need to stop using—something they may not be ready to hear.

Imagine then, the guardedness that such people feel when they are placed on an inpatient dual-diagnosis unit. They face the conflict of holding out hope that hospitalization or even therapy can provide an answer while their instinct tells them to run, hide, and somehow pretend the nightmare is not happening. Not knowing which feeling is true feeds their lack of trust, and this, then, remains a barrier to the treatment provider as well as the patient. Unfortunately, it is difficult to trust in an environment where others seem very different from oneself. People who suffer from depression may feel out of place and anxious if they are in a unit filled with patients who have acute mental illness. Some patients are sicker than others, and this difference is felt most acutely by the patients, who are nonetheless required to form the semblance of a community.

One of the requirements for admission to our dual-diagnosis unit was that individuals come to us detoxed and stabilized on their medication. People who applied for admission, or their caseworkers who called, were thoroughly informed about this. However, with the increasing difficulty in finding placements in inpatient detoxes, we often took in patients who were only hours away from their last use of drugs or alcohol, and some were homeless, unmedicated, frightened, and unable to distinguish between reality and hallucination. With patience, compassion, the right medications, and time, many were able to stay clean and sober, find medications that made them feel better, and learn about their dual diagnosis. An important part of our treatment process was referring patients on to the appropriate level of care, making sure that they have financial coverage, transportation, housing, and, most important, the motivation to become a part of a recovery community on a continuing basis.

In the following vignette, I present the story of Vincent, an individual in a treatment setting for which he is too unstable mentally. His story conveys the pain, fear, and confusion of an individual who feels separate and in danger. Vincent, despite all our ministrations, never acclimated to our inpatient unit. We moved too quickly for someone as ill as he and the methods we used were just too frightening for him. Temporarily, we were able to win Vincent's trust, only, finally, to lose it.

Vincent's paranoia manifested in auditory hallucinations (hearing voices) and in delusions (the false belief that he was being poisoned or chased). I could not immediately challenge the falsity of what he believed to be true. I had to meet him where he was. Although this helped me to gain Vincent's trust at first, this patient and I were always on shaky ground. Untrained and unequipped to deal with someone as ill as Vincent, we found ourselves unable to give him the kind of help he needed. His story is presented in the hopes that others similar to him will find the answers and safety they seek.

Vincent's Story

I first met Vincent at lunchtime on the unit. He'd just come into rehab and had been sent down to the small lunchroom where twenty-four diverse, often seriously ill patients sit down and eat together. Clearly, this was traumatic for Vincent. He cowered over by the counter where the microwave sits, as far from the other patients as he could get. His lips moved constantly in a litany of barely audible whispers to his inner voices. The tray containing his lunch sat on the serving counter, untouched.

Occasionally, we receive patients in rehab who have been without their medication for a period of time and who have been using drugs on a regular basis. Naturally, this creates some paranoia, but I had yet to see anyone react as severely as Vincent was, and I was uncertain as to what I could do to calm him.

Vincent was a Hispanic male, in his early twenties, who was extremely slender, almost emaciated. His dark hair curled around his face wildly, obscuring his features. His clothes were baggy and a foul odor emanated from his body. In every way, Vincent appeared to be trying to keep people away from him. Knowing this, I realized I would have to allow him as much space as possible.

Slowly, I walked over to him and asked him if he needed help with the microwave. I kept between us what I thought was a comfortable distance for him. He shook his head in denial and then asked me, in a breathless voice, if he could go to his room. Gesturing toward his untouched tray, I asked him if he was hungry. He gave the tray a sidelong glance, a look of terror on his face. I realized he was afraid of the food.

Reaching to the cabinets above the microwave, I brought down an unopened loaf of bread and an unopened sealed jar of peanut butter. I set these in front of Vincent and handed him a plastic knife. He took a deep breath and, without looking at me, ripped open the bread and pulled out a few slices. He inspected the peanut butter, making sure it was sealed, and then opened it and began slathering thick layers of peanut butter over the bread. Turning his back to me and the other patients, he began stuffing the dry mixture into his mouth. Afraid he might choke, I went to the refrigerator and got a handful of sealed juice boxes and brought them to him.

Knowing he'd want privacy, I returned to my seat at the serving table and watched him covertly, amazed at how much bread and peanut butter he was putting away. I could see that he had probably not been able to find food he could trust for some time. When a patient can't trust the food that he is given, he likely won't be able to trust the medication that he is given either. I doubted, watching Vincent, if we'd be able to stabilize Vincent in our rehab program, let alone offer him treatment.

After lunch, the patients left the lunchroom to line up for smoke break. I was surprised to see that Vincent had neatly put away the peanut butter and bread and had cleaned the crumbs from the counter. I stood by the counter for a moment, wondering how it would feel to be in a world such as his, where voices continually harass, warn, and denigrate, to have fear following

me everywhere, so that I could not eat or sleep or even exist with other people.

Vincent did not go down to smoke break, though I was fairly sure he
smoked. Checking his personal belongings, which were still waiting in the
nurse's station, I saw that he had not brought in any cigarettes. Stuffed into a
plastic trash bag was a mix of half-clean and half-dirty clothes, along with a
backless paperback Bible. I had wondered if Vincent was literate and supposed this meant he was.

I was certain by now that Vincent's diagnosis would be paranoid schizophrenia. As I read through Vincent's scanty records, I saw that a case management team had brought Vincent in for treatment. He'd had no detox, was
given no money or cigarettes, and possessed inadequate clothing. Vincent
had been frequenting an inner-city drop-in center and had come to the attention of a caseworker who had hoped that we would be able to get him off
drugs and back on his medication. Vincent had given little information about
himself to the caseworker. Records showed that he'd been in and out of the
state psychiatric hospital three times in the past year. His family, the records
revealed, would have nothing to do with him. When he was not in the hospital, he wandered the streets, vulnerable and sick.

Where to start? I peeked into Vincent's room and saw that he'd burrowed
into his bed. For the time being, I left him there. I wanted to speak with others
on the treatment team about the best way to approach Vincent. His apparent
paranoia made it difficult for me to decide how to engage him.

Late that afternoon, all of us involved in Vincent's care discussed how we
would manage his treatment. He'd already refused all medication since
coming onto the unit, and it appeared as if he intended to hide in his bed for
as much of the time as possible. If we were even to begin to engage him,
he'd have to be less paranoid; for that to happen, he would have to be on
medication, which he was refusing.

The staff psychiatrist suggested that I talk to Vincent about getting back
on his medication since I'd been able, earlier, to get him to eat something. I
found Vincent in his room, still cowering under the sheets. Standing outside
his door, I spoke quietly so I wouldn't alarm him. I told him my name and
asked if I could come into the room. Slowly the sheet came down off his face
and one eye peeked out. He nodded slowly. I asked Vincent if he felt better
after having eaten. Again, the slow nod. Next, I asked him if anyone had told
him why he was at this hospital. He said briefly that he knew he was in rehab.
Slowly, he eased the sheet up and over most of his face.

Did he know what rehab was? I asked. He said, his voice trembling, that
all he knew was that he did not think he could stay. When I asked him why he
did not think he could stay, he said there were too many people and too
much noise. He said he did not feel safe. I agreed with him that this place
was noisy, but I went on to talk to him about ways we would guarantee his
safety. I told him that this was a locked unit, so unsafe people would stay out,
and I reassured him that we knew the patients who were here and we supervised them carefully.

Vincent's one eye peered at me as he whispered that he was fairly sure
someone wanted to poison him. I nodded to show him I was listening and he

went on, saying that he was afraid to eat the food or take medicine. He said he felt safe only when he was alone. I edged closer to his bed, promising Vincent that I wanted only to help him. He looked steadily at me for a few seconds, and I could almost see a ray of belief in his eyes. I reminded him about the safe food I had given him and he nodded, acknowledging that. The sheet moved down and I could see both of his eyes.

I went on to assure Vincent that we would try to get safe medicine for him too. I told him that taking medication was a part of our treatment program and that we would give him medicine that would help him to feel less afraid. He went on whispering about how he was being chased, emphasizing that he did not want to go back to the city. I asked him if he meant the city the caseworker had brought him from, and he nodded assent. Considering that Vincent might be legitimately in danger from an unpaid drug dealer, I told him that, if he completed treatment on our unit, we might arrange for him to be placed in a different area. This was more than Vincent wanted to think about at the moment, though, and he again drew his blanket over his face, signifying he was through talking.

For the next day or two Vincent subsisted on peanut butter sandwiches until we were able to order in some other sealed foods that he was sure no one else had touched. The issue of Vincent's medicine remained unresolved and he spent most of his time under the covers in his bed.

If Vincent had been any other patient, he would have been discharged the first day, but we knew that he was almost totally without support. The caseworker who had brought him was not answering his phone, and Vincent had nothing to say about where he could go, except that he did not want to go back to the city because it was not safe. We were certain that if we did discharge him, he'd be back on the street, smoking crack and more paranoid than ever. Paranoid people are targets—we all knew that. Without proper case management and some street knowledge, Vincent probably wouldn't be alive long.

Vincent began to come to some groups, finally, always sitting near the doorway so he could make a quick escape if he got too scared. Sometimes he'd say a word or two to staff or one of his peers. Vincent sidling down the halls murmuring quietly to himself, sometimes laughing at a particularly funny inner voice, became a regular sight.

After a week, our psychiatrist was able to win Vincent's trust enough for him to agree to an intramuscular injection of an antipsychotic medication. We all had high hopes that, at last, we'd get a chance to see the real Vincent underneath the psychosis. I had visions of engaging him in treatment, finally, and being able to teach him some ways of surviving with his illness.

The morning after Vincent had received his injection, the first thing I saw was Vincent, hair wild around his face, eyes clenched in rage, pacing rapidly up and down the hall. He'd get to one end, hit the wall, and swing around to pace back in the other direction. Trying to catch up with him, I asked him what was wrong. Angrily he shouted that he'd been poisoned, just as he knew he would be. From the way he could not stop moving, I suspected that he was suffering from an uncomfortable side effect of his medication: the need for constant movement. However, all he could understand at the moment was that he could not stop pacing and he was very angry. At least Vincent was not a quiet little mouse anymore, though. In the middle of his pacing, he shouted loudly that he wanted to leave and he wanted to leave *now!*

We called Vincent's caseworker and actually reached him this time. As we told him what had happened, Vincent paced and shouted the whole time, and I was afraid we would have to put him in restraints, something we rarely do on our unit. It was a hectic two hours until Vincent's caseworker could arrive to pick him up—a time during which I thought long and hard about other, better ways we could have handled Vincent's treatment.

Now, I realized, he was more afraid of medicine than ever before and probably from now on would only ever take it in a psychiatric hospital where he was forced to take it. Unless the medication and the dosage are correct, he would always be at risk for the kind of side effects he was experiencing now. I thought of all the homeless people with schizophrenia who appear to prefer the warmth of a subway grate to that of a hospital room or boarding home. Convinced the world is not a safe place, they wander alone, cold and without destination.

As Vincent left the unit with his caseworker that afternoon, I reflected upon his being almost the exact age of my own son. What kind of future waited for him? I smiled and waved, knowing he did not want to be touched, but he averted his eyes. For a time he had trusted me and I knew, from his eyes, that I had let him down.

Fear of medication is not just confined to those who have schizophrenia, I realized, watching Vincent walk away. Medication changes us. Who are we on medication? Are we wiser or more in control? How do we know whether to take more or less or maybe a different medication altogether? Sometimes, for many of my patients, Vincent included, the answer would always be that it is easier just to get high.

Although side effects of medication can be treated or avoided, when a person lacks trust or is paranoid, it may be impossible for him or her to comply with a treatment regimen. Finding the right medication to assist a person with mental illness in being more comfortable and functional often requires more than one medication trial. Further, psychotropic medications often take several days or weeks to "kick in" and side effects are lessened. This requires patience on the part of the person taking the medication and good communication with the doctor dispensing it.

People seeking treatment for mental illness and addiction and their families need to investigate the types of medication available, their side effects, and the need for compliance with dosages. Families may believe that the treatment facility is trying to get their family member addicted to yet another drug, and they should understand the differences between addictive and nonaddictive substances. Families may also feel ashamed or embarrassed that their family member has to be on medication. They may blame themselves or think they failed as parents or caregivers. Families should receive ongoing support and perhaps consider therapy to learn to cope with their family member's illness and need for medication.

The role of family members (or some strong support system) becomes particularly important when a person with a mental illness is too ill to make appropriate decisions for himself (as Vincent was). When family members are frightened of or angry with an individual who may have been acting out in mental illness or addiction, they can become lacking in the motivation, energy, and courage necessary to make treatment decisions.

However, today we have many successful treatment options for people with mental illness and addiction problems. Finding these treatment options, trusting someone to administer them, and having the patience and the faith to engage in and trust the process is, for many, the most difficult part. Those who find themselves in this position may find it necessary to consider the progressive nature of mental illness and addiction. For many who do not receive treatment, their life losses will continue to increase as their quality of life decreases. As difficult as it may be to build trust with treatment providers and in medication regimens, letting mental illness and addiction progress can have a tragic end.

Chapter 3

Misunderstandings About Dual Diagnosis

Many behaviors common with mental illness and addiction are difficult to understand. A familiar saying in group meetings is, "The definition of insanity is doing the same thing over and over again and expecting, each time, different results." This refers, of course, to the addict's inability to see his or her substance abuse in a realistic way. Where drinking or drug abuse is concerned, the addict remains in denial—of alienating people, of damaging personal health, of creating financial distress, and of the actual dependence on the substance that he or she may have formed.

Denial is a primary part of the disease of addiction. Addicts often seem, to their families and people who know them, incredibly uncomprehending about what their substance abuse is doing to them and to those around them. In working with addicts who are seeking recovery, I often hear them say that they cannot themselves understand their own denial about substance abuse, and because of this they must remain cautious in recovery. Thus, the need arises, in twelve-step programs, for continuing meetings, supportive mentors, and service to others who are in addiction.

People who are not addicted may never fully understand the addict's denial, especially when the person may have been in recovery for years and, seemingly for no reason, slips back into the addiction again. The denial manifested by addicts contributes to the stigma addicts experience within the general population. If people will not admit how seriously ill they are, often friends and family interpret this as an irresponsible stance on the part of the addicts. They may be seen as people who are persisting in a lazy or unproductive lifestyle because they are "too lazy to stop." Dually diagnosed people must cope with not only the stigma attached to addiction but also the long-prevailing misunderstandings about people with mental illness.

I work with people who tell me, "You have no idea what it is like to hear your family admit that they are afraid of you." Family members do sometimes fear the person who has a mental illness. They may not know how to cope with the person's unpredictability, sometimes bizarre behaviors, or ongoing neediness.

For many years, people thought that psychiatric hospitals were the only place for people with mental illness. Some people still think this today. They may have little knowledge of the newer psychotropic medications that now allow even severely mentally ill patients to live productive and satisfying lives outside the hospital.

I often hear parents comment that they know the mental illness their son or daughter has was not inherited from them: "It was a result of all that drugging." Although using drugs and/or alcohol can damage an already fragile psyche, it is not usually the cause of mental illness. However, it is still common to hear people say, "He brought it on himself" or "She brought it on herself."

In numerous cases, the symptoms of the mental illness can be the impetus for the individual to begin drug or alcohol use as a kind of self-medication. However, even the self-medicating individual can eventually end up addicted. The reason why a person begins substance abuse does not dictate whether the individual becomes an addict.

Symptoms of dual diagnosis may be difficult for individuals and their families to understand, tolerate, and control. For example, in compulsion, the individual may feel compelled to perform certain behaviors and be unable to resist. However, family members may think the individual is behaving this way to get attention, to act out, or to embarrass them. Friction in the family results, then, and the mentally ill person may be scapegoated or avoided.

In this chapter, I address some troublesome behaviors, reasons for those behaviors, and ways of coping with them. Again, my main purpose is to assist dually diagnosed individuals and their families in understanding that acceptance of these two diseases is possible and necessary. Before acceptance can come, understandably, denial, bargaining, and grieving—but acceptance precedes wellness and wholeness.

First, I will focus on abnormal versus normal behavior. If we examine other cultures or even this culture in different times, we find that behaviors which are thought of as normal today would have been seen as bizarre twenty-five years ago such as teenagers tossing one another around in mosh pits or people of all ages walking, driving, and eating while talking on cell phones. *Normal* is relative to the time, place, and, most of all, perspective of the person who is viewing the behavior. Appropriate education about addiction and mental illness can assist individuals and their families in forming an appropriate perspective regarding what to expect. Support groups, aftercare programs, case managers, psychiatrists, and counselors can provide this education on a continuing basis.

Support groups can help individuals sort through the behaviors that can be affected by psychotropic medications and those which may be a part of the essential nature of the dually diagnosed person. These groups can assist individuals and family members in learning ways of most effectively communicating with respect and patience. Support groups can intercede, when necessary, at times when fears and emotions get out of control and individuals feel unsupported and unappreciated.

We are long past the time when families used to shut away their mentally ill relatives and lie about their illness. Today, understanding of what mental illness is and how it can be treated is increasing daily. This knowledge is there for the taking and dually diagnosed individuals no longer need to feel ashamed of being "different." Hopefully, the stories in this chapter will shed light on how it feels to "walk in someone else's shoes."

WHAT IS "NORMAL" VERSUS "ABNORMAL" BEHAVIOR?

The following vignette presents Craig, an individual who suffers from obsessive-compulsive disorder (OCD). Craig felt that to act normal he had to sedate himself, thereby hoping to act and appear more similar to others. Unfortunately, it was this very self-medicating that caused him to fall into addiction and, finally, more life unmanage-ability.

Craig's Story

My new client had a pressing question for me. He'd barely sat down for our interview when he suddenly needed to know if my office had a bathroom. Trying to set him at ease, I suggested that he go back to his room for a moment and use his own bathroom. Smiling shyly, my client assured me he did not want to *use* a bathroom; he just wanted to get a look at mine. Before I could comment, he slipped out of his chair and opened the door to the small bathroom adjoining my office and peered in at it.

I had not known Craig well enough at that point to be aware that a major obsession he lived with was a need to "check" any and every bathroom in his immediate vicinity. It was never clear to me what role Craig's bathroom checking played, but I found, early on, that it would be a major obstacle to his comfortably receiving treatment in our rehab program.

Shortly, Craig returned to his chair and began to share with me about his reasons for coming into rehab. In every way he seemed like a perfectly normal guy, affable even as he spoke of his recent loss of his job as an evening security guard because of his excessive drinking and sedative use. His supervisor had caught him sleeping one time and had requested a urine drug screen. Craig said he had felt discriminated against since many of the other security guards caught a nap now and then and weren't tested for drug use. When his urine drug screen had come back positive, he had been terminated from the job.

Craig went on to tell me that he viewed his drinking and use of sedatives as a necessity if he were to hold onto a job or even a decent relationship. In the middle of telling me this, he got out of his chair and headed for my bathroom again. He stood in the bathroom door a few moments, and then returned to his seat. He told me then that he knew some of his behaviors were strange but he couldn't help them. He insisted that, sober, he had almost no control over his obsessive behaviors, such as "checking" bathrooms. He said that people usually thought he was strange and his knowledge of how they were viewing him made his behaviors worse.

Craig said that some of his other compulsions were common ones, such as checking stove burners, counting things, washing his hands, and performing senseless rituals, such as untangling fringe on rugs or lining up articles on tabletops. As he spoke, I noticed that he had put most of the articles on his side of my desk in a neat row. I knew, talking to Craig, that I'd have to be patient and uncritical about his drinking and his mental illness. He'd made it clear that others in his life thought he had more of a problem than he thought he did.

In his early thirties, Craig had been reduced to living at home with his parents since his job loss. His parents had not been aware, until they saw Craig daily, how much tolerance to alcohol he'd built up, nor had they been aware of the exacerbation of his OCD. Craig expressed anger at his family's lack of understanding, stressing that they just wanted the rehab to "fix" him. By the time we'd finished the intake, Craig had "checked" my bathroom four times and had my desk shipshape! I felt that he had given me only a superficial sense of who he was, mainly because he was so defensive, the OCD complicating my inability to connect with Craig. It was as if there'd been three people in the room: me, Craig, and the OCD.

Craig's records gave me the information that he had been an anxious, insecure person for much of his life. His father was a high-ranking military officer, now in retirement, and he'd been demanding with Craig, Craig's mother, and the one other child in the family, his sister, now twenty-five. The family had a history of moving around the country on a regular basis. Craig had been in at least eight schools, had made few friends, and had graduated with barely average grades. Although Craig had flunked out after two semesters in community college, his sister had graduated from a well-known university and was now completing her law degree.

Craig had found his niche in night watchman work and had finally made a barely tolerable existence for himself in his own apartment where he'd drink or sleep during his spare time and work the rest of the time. Only now, since everything had fallen apart for him, had Craig's dysfunction become painfully visible to his parents, particularly Craig's father who had little patience for such blatant failure to thrive.

By Craig's own admission, many of his compulsions came from a need to "feel safe." Many people with OCD report that they feel a temporary relief from anxiety when they perform one of their rituals. Often, though, the source of the "unsafe" feeling is the real riddle. Does it stem from an abusive childhood, poor self-esteem, or performance anxiety, or is it merely an issue of brain chemistry?

With the development of SSRIs (antidepressants that address serotonin imbalance in the brain) clinicians have seen success treating some people with OCD. After maintaining compliance on a certain dose of an SSRI antidepressant for a few weeks, clients might report a reduction of symptoms. Though this form of treatment may never provide the answer to the origin of the "unsafe" feelings that cause the compulsions, it can provide relief for many, if the SSRI is the appropriate one for the individual, if the dosage is correct, and if the individual is compliant on the medication. As a therapist I have always been torn between the desire to get to the root of what causes a symptom while also wanting the patient to experience relief from the symptom as soon as possible. Our staff psychiatrist espoused a belief in the need for medication first and foremost. Though we probably couldn't get a therapeutic level of the SSRI in three weeks' time, we could get Craig off to a good start.

In the days ahead, Craig and I got to know each other well, if only through his consistent interest in my bathroom. He'd make his way up and down the halls of the rehab several times a day, ducking in and out of patients' rooms and bathrooms, "checking." I'd get a breathless "Hi" and a glimpse of Craig's sheepish face as he'd quickly duck into my office and turn slightly for a sighting of my bathroom. I'd usually try to leave the door ajar for him to save him time and embarrassment.

Even on his new medication, Craig was still "checking," and I was puzzled as to how to help him begin to talk about his feelings. One thing was clear from the beginning, and that was how thoroughly Craig's behaviors served to alienate him from his peers. They did not understand why Craig felt it necessary to look at their bathrooms on a regular basis and became quite unpleasant about his visits. Craig and I spoke about how torn he felt between his desire to form relationships or to give in to his compulsions. He was quite aware of how annoyed others were by his rituals, and he'd made efforts in his life to work this out. He said that he had chosen night jobs for this very reason, since people had difficulty tolerating his behaviors.

It was clear Craig thought he would never change. It was as if he were a prisoner of some inner force that made him do things he had not chosen. Or had he? As I got to know Craig better, he began to speak more about his father and how nothing he'd ever done had been enough to please his father. He spoke angrily about the rude awakening his sister was in for if she thought their father would settle for her becoming a lawyer. He was sure his dad would want her to be a judge or some high-ranking political figure. When I asked Craig what he had thought his father's expectations had been of him, he, smiling apologetically, stated that, as a bona fide "screwup," he had managed to get himself out of the running early on. When I asked whether he believed he was a screwup, he was quiet a moment and then admitted that maybe he had beat his father at his own game. He laughed, saying that his father would be happy now if Craig could just stay sober.

What might happen, I asked, if the medication we were giving Craig worked and he got on top of his addiction and his OCD? Craig pointed out to me how much he was still checking bathrooms. He assured me the medication would not work. I reminded Craig that I had seen him checking only twice the day before, and that perhaps the medication was beginning to help him. Craig was speculative, a whole new way of thinking was opening up to him. He asked me if he might begin to be similar to "everybody else." When I told him he might, he spoke aloud about how much time he would finally have in a day without his compulsions—time to do what he wanted to do and not what his compulsions demanded. He was silent for a long interval. He sat, absently fingering my gold desk clock, seemingly transfixed by the wagging pendulum.

Finally, I spoke. I asked Craig what kind of relationship he might have with his father if he were a normal guy—clean and sober, no compulsions, and finally able to control his behaviors. Craig remained silent, a troubled expression on his face. We'd come to a moment that was very familiar to me. No matter how ill a person is, almost always, finally, an element of secondary gain comes from this long period of suffering. Wellness very likely will cause a loss, and often a person realizes this, even if only subconsciously. I've seen many patients, at this juncture, close the door on the option of getting well, as it feels too risky.

In a low voice, Craig finally said that not being the screwup in his father's eyes would be something he couldn't even imagine. He did not know how it would feel for him. I nodded, acknowledging the confusion and fear I'd heard. Then I asked Craig to think about what we had just talked about and told him

I would see him again the next day. He bolted out of my office, clearly relieved to go. After he'd left, I thought about how invested we become in the routines of our life, even the dysfunctional ones. I thought, too, of how much easier it is to choose failure than to succumb to it on someone else's terms.

By the end of the week, it was clear that Craig was responding favorably to the SSRI he'd been prescribed. His incidents of checking had diminished appreciably and he was finally beginning to form some friendships among his peers. With Craig's consent, I scheduled a family meeting with Craig and his parents on the upcoming Saturday. I asked Craig if he felt able to express some of the feelings we'd been discussing in therapy with them in that meeting. He admitted it would be difficult for him, but he would give it a try.

Throughout the remaining days of treatment, Craig opened up more and more to me in individual therapy. We talked increasingly about his addiction and of his need to know that, even though he'd used liquor to self-medicate, he was still an alcoholic and would need to participate in a twelve-step program. Craig verbalized an insight that the addiction along with the compulsion had created walls between himself and others. He admitted that, sober and on the right medication, he would have to learn much about the proper way to relate to others. He said, too, that he was not sure he had the courage for it. I asked Craig whether he wanted the "walls" to come down. He responded that sometimes he did and sometimes he did not. It was a frightening proposition, we both agreed, and one that would take time for Craig and support from many sources.

I'd wanted a commitment from Craig because I knew he had a lot of work ahead of him to change his behaviors on an ongoing basis. We spoke about cognitive-behavioral therapy, which he would need to commit to in aftercare. This therapy gradually exposes a client to the thoughts underlying compulsions. Gradually, Craig would learn that he will be "safe" if he reduces and eventually eliminates these behaviors and thoughts. In combination with the medication he was on, this therapy would give Craig a good chance at changing, but I wanted him to know that he would have to be (and remain) willing to change. We also discussed a number of support groups he could go to after discharge in addition to AA.

When Craig's father and mother came in to meet with us on Saturday, his mother revealed to us, early in the session, that she'd suffered from panic attacks since Craig's infancy. We discussed how panic disorder is related to OCD in that the person is responding to a thought that is real to him or her even though it may not be based in reality. Craig and his mom were able to discuss some thoughts and feelings they'd never talked about before, and they both admitted that they were beginning to understand that inherited brain chemistry was probably responsible for their shared behaviors.

Craig's father, who had not said much at the beginning of the session, toward the end, questioned the role that his being so demanding had played in his son's and in his wife's behaviors. Craig did not wait for me to answer the question. He told his dad that it had not been easy living with someone who seemed ready to explode all the time. His father digested that for a moment and then admitted that, in the past, he had not thought Craig and his mother had been trying very hard, and it really had angered him at times. He acknowledged that he had been learning a lot in the past few weeks from some outpatient counseling he and his wife had been receiving while Craig was in the hospital. He was now willing to reassess the negative effects of his own behavior on these two sensitive individuals whom he loved very much. With some humility, he admitted that he was now beginning to realize that people could be trying hard when they appeared not to be and that, as he was getting older, he was realizing the need for more tolerance and patience on his part.

It was gratifying to me to hear this admission from Craig's father and, judging by the expressions on Craig's and his mom's faces, I imagined they were frankly amazed by it. In any case, it was clear we'd made a start at gaining some new perspectives in this family, and it was more than I could possibly have hoped to achieve in just one session. Our time was up for that day, but I felt positive about our progress, as I ushered Craig and his family into another room where they could talk a little longer before saying "good-bye." Once again, I'd seen a patient decide to connect instead of remaining behind his wall of illness. I did not know if Craig would follow up in outpatient care. I did know, however, that he'd given up the notion that he was hopeless, and it sounded as if his parents had too.

It is clear from this vignette that Craig's father's perspective on Craig's illness had played an important role in the past and would remain significant in the future as Craig continued in recovery. Behaviors of Craig's that had been unfathomable and maddening to his father could now be seen as symptoms of an illness that Craig had been suffering alone with for some time. Not all families come to an acceptance and understanding of the symptoms and behaviors accompanying mental illness as quickly as Craig's family did. Habits that have prevailed over many years are difficult to break. Sometimes families become invested in having someone to blame and scapegoat and they are unwilling to change this.

Much freedom from suffering comes when all members of a family become willing to receive education and deepen understanding regarding the illness of a family member. Positive thinking breeds positive action and the potential for growth for all. Craig's checking, his OCD, and his addiction may be controlled by compliance with a strict treatment plan on Craig's part, but the willingness to change perspective exhibited by his father represents something that only Craig's father could have chosen to do—to react with sensitivity and compassion. It is my hope that family therapy could always have this kind of result, for the benefit of the patient who is a part of that family, but, most important, for the benefit of the family as a whole.

HOW IS MY GRANDIOSITY A PROBLEM?

In psychiatry, grandiosity is generally defined as a person's having an exaggerated sense of his or her own importance that sometimes reaches delusional proportions. Though we may have acquaintances who irritate us with their tendency to be self-focused or to take themselves too seriously, encounters with people who are truly grandiose tend to be infrequent.

A cultural tradition that we are often taught, from childhood, is not to brag about ourselves, build ourselves up too much, or put ourselves first before others. People who act and speak as if they are superior to others can be disconcerting to us, and if this is a typical behavioral pattern, we will probably simply avoid them after a while. However, when formerly mild-mannered, quiet people suddenly become pushy, vociferous, and argumentative, those who know and love them may be at a loss as to how to respond.

Spouses of alcoholics regularly experience this type of personality change when their spouses drink too much. Other drugs, such as cocaine, amphetamines, and hallucinogens, can also change a person's personality in a rapid and puzzling way. It is difficult for family members to endure ongoing personality changes that may occur in their addicted family members. For this reason, families may live in fear of the substance abusers and of who they are when using. The addict's spouse and children never know from one day to the next how the person may behave, and because addiction is a family system disease, everyone in the family is affected by this unpredictable way of life. This fear and discomfort is compounded for the family members of the person who is dually diagnosed because such personality changes may be more severe with mood swings or paranoia, or some other symptom of active mental illness.

Many kinds of personality changes can be manifested in individuals depending on the kind of mental illness present, and I will not attempt to describe them all here. What I want to examine instead is how these ongoing personality changes feel for the people who experience them and for their friends and families. What can be done to get through them? Do medications help? Does arguing help? Does setting boundaries and showing tough love help?

To begin to fathom ways of dealing with personality changes, especially grandiosity, we must first examine the reaction of the people who experience the personality change. Many individuals I have worked with have said they sought courage and the ability to be assertive when drinking or using drugs. When they became sober, they did not know how to deal with their own meek, shy personality. For these individuals, being aware of anger and being able to express it may not have been possible unless they were drinking or using drugs. Then, perhaps, volcanic rages may have erupted each time they were under the influence, perhaps even in a blackout. Sober, they might not even remember or believe what occurred in their rage.

For such people to learn how to live soberly in a family environment, they must become willing to explore how to experience their feelings and to express them to others in sobriety. They must regain credibility with family members who may have feared and avoided them for years. For people who are abstinent and in recovery from an addiction, grandiose or rageful behaviors can change with their (and their families') agreement to pursue family therapy, which will address new ways of communicating and experiencing feelings.

For dually diagnosed individuals, the process is more complicated. For instance, individuals with bipolar disorder, who experience mood swings that are triggered by their brain chemistry and stressors, may enter a "manic" phase wherein they become overactive, talkative, sleepless, and busy. They may have experienced manic phases before and may, in fact, look forward to them as times of increased creativity. They may not be interested in how these behaviors affect their family members, who are, during the mania, subjected to their nocturnal roamings, rushed and impatient speech, and argumentativeness. Further, they may resent being told by their family members that they are "sick" and need to be on medication.

In my work with dually diagnosed individuals, I have met many people with bipolar disorder who were being diagnosed for the first time at midlife. For years, these individuals may have used alcohol to "take the edge off" the mania so that they could sleep or experience thoughts that did not race in their minds. For years, they may have experienced, after periods of mania, crushing depression that they would also seek to self-medicate with alcohol or perhaps cocaine. When first discovering they have a mood disorder, they might at first be relieved to discover that mood stabilizers can help them get off the roller coaster of mood swings. However, after months of experiencing normal moods, they might report that they miss their manic periods and that the medication makes them feel bored and unlike them-selves.

Even though people may remain engaged in recovery from their addiction, going to AA meetings and remaining abstinent, they might begin to resist taking the mood stabilizer that had at first seemed to be a lifesaver. Families who saw their dually diagnosed family members improve on this "magic" pill that evened out the moods, making life so much easier for everyone, may, understandably, become angry and disappointed when they stop taking their medication and resume old behaviors—perhaps even returning to addictive behaviors. Just as alcoholics may wish to moderate their drinking some day, so people with mental illness may harbor hopes that they can go off medications after a time and be normal. It is essential that dually diagnosed individuals and their families work closely with a psychiatrist on an ongoing basis to establish and maintain medication compliance. A psychiatrist who comes to know these individuals, their habits and stressors, should be the only person to make decisions about how to adjust medication dosages.

The vignette that follows tells the story of Allan, who was experiencing a manic episode while in our rehab program. Our efforts to educate Allan about the dangers inherent in not taking his medication were unsuccessful. Lost in euphoria, he felt invincible. The vignette reveals the tragedy inherent in untreated mental illness, not only for the patient but also for those whom he or she loves.

Allan's Story

Allan was flying high when he came to rehab. Diagnosed bipolar, Allan admitted to having been off his medication for several weeks, and he appeared manic. A blackjack dealer in one of our nearby casinos, Allan had lost control on the job, interrupting his dealing with loud discourses on how he could win any and all games he dealt. "The dealer reigns supreme!" he'd been heard to shout from his post behind the blackjack table one night, and it wasn't long before he'd been led off by security staff in front of a tableful of disgruntled gamblers.

Allan had been taken to a local crisis center where routine blood and urine tests revealed high levels of methamphetamines, cannibis, and alcohol in his system. Records showed that Allan had a history of hospitalizations for manic episodes. Because of his substance abuse issues, Allan had been sent to us for stabilization on medication and for education about dual-diagnosis issues. What Allan's records did not show, however, was that he was also a sex addict, especially active when in the manic phase of his illness. This we would find out later in some very uncomfortable ways.

Allan was admitted at around five o'clock on a Friday, an awkward time for me to receive new clients, because I am unable to fully engage with them until the following Monday. Because the addictions counselor serves as a primary advocate for the patient, the patient who has not been engaged by a counselor may feel "high and dry" for a time.

I took a few moments on my way off the unit that afternoon to introduce myself to Allan, who had set up camp outside the nurses' station. He'd begun a running dialogue with the two nurses who were there, stepping in and out of the glass enclosure to wave his hands around close to their faces to emphasize his points. Despite repeated requests from the nurses, Allan would not stop talking nor would he go to his room. I could see from the expressions on their faces that they were quickly running out of patience with him.

Seeing me, Allan turned away from the nurses and began bitterly complaining that everyone had been telling him to come back "later," and he guessed I'd be saying the same thing to him. He paced back and forth around me as he spoke, too busy or preoccupied to meet my eyes. I told Allan that I was his counselor and could talk to him for a few minutes if he wished. Allan swiveled his head rapidly and gave me a discomfiting up-and-down assessment, then followed me to my office, where he remained standing.

I observed that he seemed restless and asked if there was anything staff could do to make Allan more comfortable. Pacing around my small office, he loudly asked me to see if I could get him out of this place. He emphasized that he was a successful guy, a top dealer in a prominent casino for the past five years. He proudly told me he had a luxury apartment and was able to attract any girl he wanted. He asked me if I didn't think that was a pretty good track record for someone only thirty-five years old. Without stopping to take a breath, he continued to stress that his using drugs was no big deal—that everyone in his line of work used drugs, mainly to stay awake. He also wondered why everyone thought his talking too much had been inappropriate. He believed it was a plus to get to know the people at his blackjack table—especially the pretty women.

Finally I managed to interrupt him—the only real tactic a therapist can use when faced with the kind of pressured speech Allan was exhibiting—and he stopped midstride. I asked him if he was saying he believed he did not need to be in rehab. I wanted to gauge the level of his denial and determine whether we would be able to get his cooperation in treatment. Disregarding my question, Allan began talking again about how he had been "dragged into" the program by people who said they "cared." Shrugging, he said he probably did need to lay off the pharmaceuticals for a while though, since they seemed to be messing up his mind—and his performance sometimes, too, he added with a wink.

So, vaguely, Allan was committing to stay, and I did believe that a weekend of stabilizing might be good for him. Maybe his medications would begin to work, he would begin detoxing, and, by Monday, I'd get a glimpse of the Allan beneath all this activity. I spent a few moments familiarizing Allan with the program's rules and our expectations, though he was too busy pacing around my office to take in much, and then I left for the weekend.

Monday morning I was met by the charge nurse, Sandy, who was very upset. Immediately, she told me Allan had to go. Then she directed me to the notes various staff had made regarding Allan's behaviors throughout the weekend. According to the report, Allan had not slept the whole weekend; he had spent the days and nights pacing, haranguing the nurses at the nurses' station, and trying to "get to know" his female peers. Even more disconcerting, a few of Allan's female peers were interested in getting to know him back. He was an attractive guy, obviously financially successful, and he had a mania-supported charisma that was hard for some to resist. Shaking her head, Sandy said she was pretty sure Allan was "cheeking" his medications (holding medications under his tongue or in his cheek and spitting them out later). She emphasized that he was clearly worse than he had been a few days before, and all the medication he was being given should have taken effect by now.

About this time Allan came sauntering down the hall with a big smile on his face. He told me excitedly that he had been waiting for me to get in so he could tell me what the staff, whom he referred to as a "bunch of yo-yos," had put him through over the weekend. I sighed and led him in to my office. In my office, I began by asking Allan how he felt about his mood stabilizer. I added that I really did need for him to sit down while we talked. He sank into a chair reluctantly, complaining that everyone was always trying to calm him down and stop him in his tracks. He emphasized how great he felt and how sure he was that he did not want to take any medication that would take those good feelings away. When asked whether he thought that was the purpose of a mood stabilizer, he gave me an irritated look and said he was sure that the staff wanted calm patients and that was probably our main reason for giving mood stabilizers. He added that he thought he and the other patients were a bunch of guinea pigs with whom we were experimenting.

Trying to remain patient, I asked Allan what he thought would happen if he let his manic mood run its full course without taking any medication at all. Shaking his head, he said he supposed, with my training, I'd know that he was going to get depressed when the mania passed. He'd experienced that many times, he said, but he knew how to get his hands on "uppers" easily enough. I reminded Allan that he'd said he wanted to lay off drugs just a few days before. Why was he here? Allan was lost to me by then, though, as he began arguing that all of us counselor types were the same—always trying to get in the last word. He stood up, ready to move on.

Firmly, I reminded Allan that if he did want to remain in rehab he was going to need to comply with his medication regimen. I told him he could not refuse it and he could not "cheek" it. I asked if what I had said to him was clear, realizing that, at this point, there really was no engaging someone at Allan's level of grandiosity. Standing by the door, and clearly eager to leave, he nodded, asking me if we were finished. Before dismissing him, I informed him that if he became romantically involved with any female peers he would be discharged. This is called setting limits, my least favorite part of counseling, but often the most necessary.

Allan was put on a liquid mood stabilizer, which he could not cheek, and he was asked to sign a contract agreeing to be appropriate in his relationships with his female peers. Surprisingly, he accepted all this and was willing to remain on the unit. After a few days, Allan began to come down from his mania and I was able to engage with him on a deeper level. In one session, he confided in me how much he dreaded the end of his mania. He spoke of how he would always be left with debt, legal charges, lost jobs, and, worst of all, the feelings of being ashamed of all he had done while manic.

I began to educate Allan, now that he was more focused, on the ability of a mood stabilizer to even out his moods so that he would not have to dread the consequences of his extreme moods. He asked me to explain how the medication could cause this "leveling out" of his moods. I reminded Allan of how manic he had been when he first came on the unit, stressing that, often, the higher the peak, the worse the crash later. Avoiding the huge peaks in mood could help Allan to avoid the serious crashes. Seeing that Allan was following what I said to him, I explained the medicine's effect on his brain and gave him some materials to read before our next session. I also encouraged him to discuss these ideas with our staff psychiatrist when they next met.

Allan accepted the reading materials but honestly admitted that he was not sure he wanted to give up his manic episodes, even if he had to suffer through the ensuing depressions. He spoke earnestly of how, when manic, he felt he could do anything or be anybody he wanted to be. I asked Allan if he had any idea how he actually appeared to other people when in a manic state. I pointed out all the losses he had experienced following his manic episodes. Allan looked doubtful, and I knew I had to give him time to think about this. His denial was strong; he wanted very badly to believe he could keep the manic periods that felt so good, despite their negative consequences.

For the next day I asked him to list some losses he'd experienced during some of his past manic episodes. By the following week, Allan and I were beginning to make some progress. He'd discussed the loss of judgment he experienced when manic and had begun to accept, he said, the increasing calmness he was feeling on his mood stabilizer.

Then came Celine. Nineteen and flawlessly beautiful, Celine was a dancer who had gotten hooked on heroin and had come to us to learn something about her diagnosis of histrionic personality disorder. She quickly became the star of the unit. Off heroin for the first time in months, she was languorously coming awake to her own beauty and to her ability to control those around her with her sexuality.

Allan was smitten. He followed Celine around like a pull toy on a string. In group, he sat near her; on smoke break, he hovered at her elbow; in the hall, between groups, he hung on her every word, mesmerized. Allan could not have been any more lost to me if someone had shot him up on methamphetamines. He was in his addiction and there was no fighting it.

By Celine's second day on the unit, Allan began refusing his mood stabilizer. I called him in to process his refusal. He reminded me that he did not like the way the medication made him feel, and it was clear he was not going to change his mind. He was eager to be out of my office and back to Celine. I reminded Allan of the treatment contract he had signed, and he threw his hands up in disgust, telling me that the treatment team and I could decide what we wanted. He'd met someone who was right for him and he wasn't going to "screw it up" for himself by taking medicine that made him feel "like a zombie."

Allan left my office and I thought about how inadequately we are able to deal with sex addiction in our unit, and elsewhere as well. Such individuals view their sexuality as an essential part of who they are and as with Allan, they often find extra libido and confidence when manic.

In the days ahead, it became clear that Allan and Celine were mutually drawn to each other. They were careful to stay within the rules of the unit by not "pairing off," and Allan returned to taking his medication, but the work Allan was doing with me had become superficial and I knew he was just marking the time. Four days before Allan was to be discharged, he and Celine decided to sign out against medical advice.

In our last session, Allan told me he knew that he was in love with her and that this was "the real thing." I told him that he had to get to know who *he* was before he could even begin to reach outside of himself enough to love someone else. I encouraged him to stay and to let Celine finish her treatment. Allan thanked me for caring but repeated that he knew what was best for him. He held out his hand to shake mine, saying that he hoped there would be no hard feelings, and that I would wish him luck.

I shook Allan's hand, but I did not wish him luck. Addiction and mental illness are too insidious for luck to be able to make a difference. I found it difficult to believe, watching this attractive couple leave our rehab facility, that there could be anything ahead for them but happiness and success, but appearances are deceiving. When people do not have the judgment or insight to know when they are not stable, life can spiral out of control. On some level, Allan had admitted this when he was willing to review his life losses during the past years.

False positive memories won out this time, however, for Allan and for Celine. Neither Allan nor Celine were able at that time to see themselves as they actually were. Lost in the glow of perceived love they had forgotten why they had sought help and now believed the "magical thinking" they had embraced for so much of their lives was true. Allan had told me he knew that, eventually, the crash and descent into depression as well as life losses lay ahead. This time, probably, Allan would take someone else down with him.

This vignette illustrates how difficult it is for people suffering from feelings of grandiosity to want to change, especially when all their feelings tell them they are doing well. On the intellectual level, Allan knew his mood swings, left unmedicated, brought a multitude of life losses, but it was difficult for Allan to use good judgment, even about what he knew to be true. The feelings of superiority were too strong. Allan faced not just the lure of an addiction to drugs and alcohol but also the lure of a sexual addiction, addictions that were difficult for him to combat when in a manic state.

No family members came forward to speak to me about Allan's progress while he was in rehab. He had long ago broken ties with those who had cared and sought to get him to change. Perhaps the most ironic thing of all—and the hardest to understand—despite Allan's apparent behavior, inside was an Allan who really did want to change. I'd met him during the few focused sessions we had managed to have. What would it take, I wondered, for that Allan finally to emerge and take charge? Would he ever get off the merry-go-round? Or would he spin faster and faster into oblivion?

WHAT'S WRONG WITH GETTING OVER ON PEOPLE?

As a counselor, it is my job to believe people unless I see evidence that what they are telling me may not be true. It is often difficult, early in treatment, to know if people are telling the truth. When I first worked with the people who came to our dual-diagnosis unit and I heard heartbreaking stories daily, I usually could not bring myself to challenge the truth of those stories. I had always believed that individuals should learn to see themselves as people who have the power to affect their destiny in a positive way. Now, a few years down the road in my counseling career, I have come to understand that individuals with addictions will often, perhaps unwittingly, use their life events to justify continuing in addiction. If addicts choose to see themselves as victims, they may well remain victims.

Counselors working with dually diagnosed individuals will find themselves pursuing several objectives. First of all, the patients seek and need validation. At the same time, though, the counselors must see to it that the individuals move along in the healing process, if possible. If the individuals fall back into self-pity or a sense of hopelessness, they risk returning to the addictive process. Seeking a balance between these goals, I have teetered, at times, more in the direction of wanting to focus on a person's need for validation. Therefore, when working with an individual who is difficult to like, someone who is cocky or shows little or no remorse, I have been known to push harder to understand those behaviors and to empathize with what may have been their origin.

For this reason, I have had some difficulty, as do many counselors, working with individuals who have been diagnosed with a personality disorder. Many personality-disordered individuals develop intricate techniques for protecting themselves from intimacy. Having suffered rejection and abandonment, many become quite adept at abandoning others in a number of subtle and maddening ways. Families, friends, and spouses of people who have personality disorders often report to me that their loved ones slip through their lives like quicksilver— there one moment and gone the next.

Understanding why individuals show symptoms of a personality disorder is difficult. Because the source is usually a poor sense of self individuals are often plagued by a lack of coping skills for dealing with life, may have limited interpersonal skills, and may see themselves as victims. They may mask this perception under a veneer of grandiosity and arrogance that keeps others at a safe distance from them, particularly if they have suffered trauma. Addiction becomes the wall that personality-disordered individuals build around themselves to keep others out. Even when their lives are at stake, when they can no longer get high, when all options are exhausted, still they may fight learning to connect with anything other than a substance.

When family members, friends, teachers, or counselors begin to establish a sense of closeness with people who have a personality disorder, a common response is to do something to push family members away—because the closeness may feel disturbingly similar to an old invasion of boundaries that has remained unhealed. One way of pushing away people who come too close is through control, and this control is exemplified by the behavior of "getting over on people."

Working on an inpatient unit, I was more than familiar with patients who tried to "get over on staff." Phone privileges, smoke breaks, extra time for counseling sessions—all were fair game. Usually, though, this was not necessarily a symptom of much more than the desire to survive and get through rehab. However, for individuals with some personality disorders, "getting over on someone" is an important and often-used coping mechanism.

This is particularly true of individuals diagnosed with antisocial personality disorder. Rather than letting these individuals "get over" or bend rules in any way, successful counselors will confront the individuals' coping behaviors that keep them from connecting with their environment. This means being firm, perhaps even harsh at times, to keep individuals on track in the learning process that will be necessary for them to achieve quality of life. Counselors will need patience and strong egos, and they will need to enforce rules and boundaries on a regular basis, not only to reassure the individuals through consistency, but also to teach what is expected in reciprocal relationships.

For individuals diagnosed with antisocial personality disorder, getting over on someone represents far more than just managing to break the rules and not get caught. The power they exert in getting over on others enables them to soothe an internal sense of impotence. Often, in this process of getting over on others, personality-disordered people may be unable to sense or feel the impact they are having on others by their behaviors. They may have difficulty accepting responsibility for their actions when they feel, in reality, empty, insignificant, and powerless. The individual who is described in the following vignette exemplifies some of the points I have just discussed.

Josh's Story

Josh came to us from jail. Now and again we receive patients who come into rehab in lieu of doing jail time, and Josh was one. He'd already been in jail for two years and, during our initial interview, laughed about how he'd gotten some of the best drugs in his life while he was in jail. I was not surprised to read in Josh's records that he was diagnosed with antisocial personality disorder, but I was surprised by how charming he was. In his midthirties, Josh was a trim, handsome man with piercing blue eyes and thick blond hair. His clothes were pressed, his hair cut neatly. No one would have guessed he had just come from jail.

Josh's records had been made available to me before my first meeting with him, and I had read through them carefully, trying to glean an understanding, as I always do, of how someone can be "antisocial." I try extremely hard to see the person underneath the diagnosis. Josh had grown up in a fairly typical suburban family, the middle child of three children. His father was an insurance salesman; his mother stayed home with the children. Josh had finished high school, gotten a job in construction and married, fathering three children of his own.

Beyond all this, however, was another Josh—a Josh only hinted at in the records, but one I became acquainted with over the three weeks we worked together. To begin with, Josh had difficulty learning in school and, because of this, had been placed in special classes. Back in his schooldays, little was known about treating learning disabilities, so Josh learned early on to develop a twofold way to treat his own problem: first, he fought a lot, and, second, he found his own brand of self-medication—amphetamines. By middle school, Josh was already started on the path that would later be his downfall.

Managing to graduate from high school with barely passing grades, Josh continued to do what he had learned best. On the job, in his marriage and wherever things weren't working for him, he used brute force to get his way. By the time Josh's third child was born, he had been arrested twice for domestic violence and once for possession of illegal drugs. He had done a lot of jail time in his life and, more than anything, had learned how to use the system to get what he wanted. When I met Josh, he had not seen his three children for over three years and his wife wanted nothing to do with him. He had been out of touch with his parents and his siblings since before his last jail stay.

When Josh related all this to me, he joked about the loose security in jail and glossed over his lack of contact with his family. He said he guessed they were just fed up with him and added, with a smile, that he couldn't really blame them since he was such a "hell-raiser." I'd thought mentioning Josh's kids and asking whether he missed them would cause some show of emotion on his part, but he said seeing them had not been worth the aggravation he got from his ex-wife. He went on to talk about what a pain in the neck it had been to live with her and how he hated having to go through her to see the kids. This was one thing I noticed about Josh. Whenever I tried to get him to talk about himself, he brought up someone else. I decided just to let Josh talk and see what developed.

Our first session lasted over an hour, and when Josh was done (mostly bragging about how he'd gotten over on so many people in his life), it seemed as though I'd begun to win his trust. At the end of the session, he told me he had enjoyed talking with me and that he now believed rehab wouldn't be as bad as he'd thought. He told me he had enjoyed talking to such a "good listener," and he was looking forward to future sessions. He expressed hope that working with me would help him to change in positive ways. Being human, I swallowed the bait—typical response, I am told, to someone who is antisocial. Josh kept the control, and I let him.

Next session, right from the beginning, Josh leaned forward and told me that because he really trusted me he was going to take a chance and be really honest with me. I nodded, waiting for him to go on. Meeting my eyes in a steady gaze, he said that I had to know that he had no intention of quitting the drugs he took because there was no way he could get along without them. He went on to reveal that he knew of at least a dozen ways to clean up his urine so his probation officer would never know that he was using. He asked me what I thought about what he'd just said.

First, I confirmed that he had three years of probation ahead of him. Then I asked him why he had told me what he'd just revealed. He said he knew I wanted him to be honest and that, since our conversation the day before, he thought he could speak to me frankly about his real intentions. I affirmed that honesty is, indeed, necessary in the recovery process. I added that what Josh had just spoken about was not recovery.

Josh sat silently, assessing me, playing a cat and mouse game. He finally went on to say that if he quit using amphetamines he would be "all over the place," unable to relate to people or do his job. I asked Josh how he thought amphetamines and the other drugs he had been using had improved his life. How did he think he could change, as he had told me he wanted to do the day before, while continuing to abuse mood-altering substances? Giving me a level look, Josh said that, so far in his life, he had managed to get what he wanted, no matter what substances he had abused. Evidently my response had not been the one he was after.

I asked Josh if he had "wanted" to be in jail all the times he had been incarcerated, and whether being in this rehab now was truly what he wanted. Abruptly, Josh asked me what I was proposing, and I responded that I was proposing Josh "get with the program." I suggested he try staying sober and talking to the doctor about his symptoms. I suggested he try working with his probation officer instead of trying to get over on him. Smiling, Josh shook his head and stood up. "Session over," he said, and I knew I had done very little to get through to him. Either we played by his rules, it seemed, or we didn't play at all.

Josh did not schedule any more sessions with me that week. Finally, I approached him to remind him that he had to speak with his addictions counselor at least three times a week to meet the requirements of the program. Josh made an appointment for the next day. At the beginning of the next session, he sat in my office, arms folded over his chest, and asked what I wanted to talk about. I reminded Josh of what he had said about how he usually got whatever he wanted wherever he went. I asked him to clarify that for me because it seemed that many aspects of his life were anything but desirable.

He chuckled, saying sarcastically that I was so busy trying to "shrink" him that I couldn't even see how little what other people thought of him meant to him. He said that people expecting him to "measure up" had no effect whatsoever on him, which, in and of itself, was very freeing for him. No one else could control him because he did not care what they thought. He went on to add that he included me in that category, so whether I liked or approved of him did not really matter. When I asked him whether it was lonely living this way, he laughed, asking me if I had noticed how many friends he had on the unit.

True, people did gravitate to Josh, attracted by his nonchalant charisma. In our rehab program, Josh was pretty much "the man." In fact, he toed a fine line to keep from being reprimanded for inappropriateness with female peers, who apparently considered Josh a "catch." As Josh's counselor, I was constantly defending him to the treatment team, who saw him as a "scammer." I kept holding on to my knowledge of the tough time Josh had as a kid—his learning disabilities, his attempts to self-medicate and to defend himself. Surely this guy could be reached in some way.

True to form, Josh figured out what I wanted and gave it to me. Next session, he began by telling me that he had thought about what I had said in our last session, and he was ready to admit that he was lonely much of the time. We spent most of the session talking about Josh's failed relationships and how he knew he needed to learn not to be so controlling. I thought we were making progress.

The next morning, however, in a meeting, our psychiatrist reported a positive result from Josh's random urine test. He revealed that, not only was Josh positive for methamphetamines, but four other patients had tested positive as well. He informed us that each of the four patients had come into rehab with negative drug screens and stated that he thought someone was passing drugs on the unit, most likely Josh.

Our policy when a patient tests positive for drugs (with a repeat test to confirm) is to discharge the patient. It's a frustrating process and interrupts everybody's treatment. In the days that followed, we discharged several patients, including Josh. I never found out who had brought drugs on the unit, but looking back on all that had transpired between Josh and me, I realized that he had been telling me the truth about himself all along. Was it a cry for help? Was it a request that I not let him scam me the way he had scammed everybody else? I felt I had failed Josh by not seeing through his charming smoke screen. For me, the enigma of antisocial personality disorder remains unsolved. As a treatment provider, I will continue to study and to learn. Hopefully, Josh will find the help he needs one day.

It is tempting to say that the Joshes of the world do not really want help, so why bother? People such as Josh may believe they are happy because they prioritize keeping control, as Josh had admitted in our discussion. However, once they begin to develop reciprocal relationships, they could experience their existence in a much more positive way. Knowing this, we, as counselors, must recognize our responsibility for providing a pathway to wellness.

I would urge those who are diagnosed with personality disorders to move beyond their comfort zone and to seek and comply with therapy, despite how risky it feels. We are meant, as humans, to connect, and certain rules and laws govern our success in connecting. To remain removed from those rules and laws is to be alone. Family members of these individuals should seek good counsel and learn how to offer their consistent love and compassion, despite the hurtful behaviors exhibited by someone who routinely avoids "connecting" or any kind of genuine intimacy.

People are not their disease. People may have a disease, but more often, the disease has them. When providing care and nurturing we must be willing to search for the people behind the defenses.

WHO'S MORE SCARED OF MY ANGER, YOU OR I?

Whenever I ask people in rehab to begin to identify their feelings, usually the first recognizable feeling they identify is anger. After years of abusing substances and "not feeling," a person who is in the first few weeks of sobriety may have difficulty processing feelings, which can come rushing back, often at an alarming rate. For family members and friends of the recovering person, this emphasis on anger can come as a shock because they feel the person has no right to be angry, when they are the ones who have been suffering.

Clearly, anger is often misunderstood as a feeling, even when addiction is not involved, and especially when it is a symptom of mental illness. It is difficult for us to conceive that some people become enraged so quickly that they act out dangerously. How can they not see it coming? How can they not control their response? Might it be that they are merely selfish, immature, or just plain evil?

These are all speculations I have heard, even from counselors, about anger management problems. Probably most of the counselor burnout I have seen comes from working daily in an environment where the negative energy of anger is constantly felt and having to be addressed. However, successful counselors know that the ability to feel and express anger is an important part of recovery, of getting beneath the layers of issues that patients may be receiving treatment for in therapy.

So what *do* recovering addicts have to be angry about, and why is this the first feeling usually identified by them in treatment? First and foremost, if they intend to get and stay sober, they now become aware that they have just lost their main coping mechanism for dealing with life's difficulties. If they truly plan never to drink or use drugs again, they are going to be terribly vulnerable.

Picture the quandary faced by adults who have been using drugs and drinking since their teenage years. If this has been their main way of coping, say, for twenty years, they probably have not developed appropriate skills for dealing with negative situations. For them, drinking and drugging may have dulled the pain, and even though problems did not get solved, they always had this haven of losing themselves temporarily through substance abuse. For many addicts, though, as tolerance builds, they are no longer able to drink or drug enough to get that much-needed relief. Now, instead, they may experience the physical pain that accompanies liver or pancreatic involvement, or the fear of having to use so much heroin or cocaine that an overdose may occur. Suddenly, the haven disappears. They are told they may die if they continue to drink or take drugs. They are told they may lose their families, money, or homes. They are told they are worthless and have no self-control. They have lost respect on their jobs and in their families, and they can no longer work or relate.

So they decide to quit. By now, though, they have accumulated so many losses that maybe no one cares that they are quitting, or maybe, since they have sung this song before, no one believes them. This is often the point at which people come for rehabilitation. Straight from jail or out of the hospital after a failed suicide attempt, they come to us, stripped of their defenses, minus their self-respect and the respect of others, and robbed of the one defense that always worked for them—until it stopped working.

Often, people in early sobriety are unable to experience any kind of pleasure (this is called anhedonia). Sometimes, too, they are angry about their inability to take pleasure in the common elements of life, especially when told that, once they become sober, everything will improve. Though we try to teach that these feelings of post–acute withdrawal will wane after they learn some coping skills and their bodies begin to produce endorphins normally again, addicts want what they want when they want it. They can't stand feeling the way they do and believe that the terrible way they feel is someone else's fault, or that they need some kind of mood-altering substance in order to be able to function in their lives. When people enter a rehabilitation setting in this frame of mind, the brunt of all that pent-up anger comes rushing out, onto counselors, peers in rehab, and, most of all, the addicts themselves.

It is difficult for those of us who have learned appropriate ways to confront people with whom we are angry to understand the buildup of rage in those who have never been able to identify anger or do anything positive about it. Often, we may think they are simply indulging the rush of "going off" on someone. Too, we tend to believe that people have a right to be angry about some things and not others. We believe, on some level, that addicts should have enough remorse about all their carousing to wake up and get over it.

People who misunderstand the anger response in early recovery may never have suffered the losses and shame of having been in active addiction for a large part of their lives. They may have no sense, even when told, of the fear that comes when one's crutch is removed and one feels helpless and hopeless about the life that lies ahead. For this reason, I have found the recovering people who regularly hosted AA and NA meetings in our rehabilitation center to be, not just helpful, but essential to the recovery process. "We've been where you are," these people would say to our angry folks, "and those feelings don't last forever. Just hang in there, one day at a time."

Only recently have we begun to diagnose a mental illness called intermittent explosive disorder, in which anger is a primary symptom. This anger involves a person's inability to resist aggressive impulses, and because of this, the person may hurt someone or destroy property. Further, with this disorder, the person appears to become much more angry than the situation warrants. (Other disorders that might cause these aggressive impulses are ruled out in choosing this diagnosis.)

The following vignette provides insight into the struggles of a person who showed symptoms of intermittent explosive disorder and what it was like to work with her.

Marley's Story

My first impression of Marley was strongly influenced by the fact that she came onto our unit in shackles. In my history as a dual-diagnosis counselor, I have seen this happen only a few times, and it is usually a sign that we are in for some difficulty. In Marley's case, we had received notice that she would be in shackles, so to protect the patient from humiliation (and for reasons of confidentiality) we cleared the halls of all patients.

Marley walked through the eerily silent halls, head down, shuffling. I wanted to see her eyes, but they were hidden by her long red hair, which swung forward across her face. As she was processed by the head nurse and the mental health worker, I stood in the nurses' station watching her reaction to the people around her, assessing how to begin to engage Marley when the proper time came.

It was difficult to believe that someone with Marley's tiny stature could have been the dangerous person about whom we'd been warned days prior to her coming. She was only a few inches above five-feet tall and slender. At age thirty, she was homeless and, for all practical purposes, alone in the world. Her parents had placed her in programs for incorrigible children from the age of fourteen on, and, finally, they had, according to the records, given up on her. She had proceeded from being a ward of the state to being a ward of jails and courts.

Watching Marley stand at the nurses' station, limply submitting to our search, I was struck by her solitariness. She appeared to be looking through those around her, and even when she raised her head and I could see her intense blue eyes, she showed no response to anything that was going on around her. Even without makeup, Marley was a strikingly beautiful woman, but it was a cold beauty. Although I do not often feel afraid of a patient, there was something in Marley that I feared, standing there, and it puzzled me.

I'd read Marley's records, which had come to us from the courts days before. She had an unusual diagnosis, intermittent explosive disorder. Simply put, a patient with this diagnosis is prone to episodes of rage brought on by aggressive impulses that the patient cannot control. These episodes are not the result of a mood disorder alone, although a mood disorder may accompany intermittent explosive disorder. There are numerous theories on where the patient's rage comes from, how it may be controlled, and, especially, whether the patient is responsible for behaviors that occur during episodes of rage.

Marley had been diagnosed with bipolar disorder and was being given a mood stabilizer and an antidepressant. According to reports, these had done little to quell her violent episodes. She had come to us for medication stabilization and for treatment for marijuana and alcohol abuse.

Suddenly, Marley became animated, swinging her head from side to side, looking for someone to hear her. She yelled for a cigarette, her demands accompanied by a flurry of loud obscenities. Writing busily, the head nurse told her no staff were available to take her outside for a smoke break, and regular smoke break would not come for another two hours. On impulse, I stepped forward and quietly told the nurse I would take Marley outside to smoke if the mental health worker could monitor us.

Marley gave me an interested stare and asked who I was. I told her I was one of the counselors and that I needed her word she would not try to take off if I made an exception to the break rules. When a patient is ordered to us from jail, we are expected to maintain security and our status as a voluntary unit no longer applies. She looked amused and made some low comment about how if she *did* run, none of us would ever catch her. She noted too that the weather outside was much too cold for a jailbreak.

Outside, I led Marley to the smoking area, lit her cigarette for her, and sat down beside her. She puffed busily, pulling her jacket collar around her ears and ignoring me. When she had almost finished the cigarette, I asked her to come to my office to talk with me once we were back inside. Staring at the bare trees around the smoking area, she mumbled that there was nothing to talk about. Then she added that I might as well know that she planned to do as little as possible in rehab since she'd come here only in lieu of going to jail.

After I had let some silent time go by, I told Marley that her decision not to engage in treatment was her choice, but I did plan to call her probation officer as soon as we got back on the floor. He would then see to it that Marley was transported to a venue where she would not be required to engage in treatment—jail. Irritated, Marley challenged me as to why I would do such a thing. I told her that our voluntary program was for people who intended to learn something about their addiction and mental illness. Clearly, if Marley did not want to show an interest in learning these things, then she did not belong here.

Marley said I was beginning to "tick her off." Rising from the bench, she glared down at me, and the mental health worker quickly joined us at the bench. I stood my ground, rising and ushering Marley toward the door back to the unit. In the elevator, she cursed steadily, and when the doors opened, she turned to me and muttered that she would come to my office after she had disposed of her jacket.

Sitting in my office waiting for Marley, I recalled the fear I'd felt when I'd first seen her. I realized at that moment that the fear I'd experienced was closely tied to Marley's own fear. People with anger problems never know what is going to happen to them and any unpleasantness that does happen is usually a result of their own actions. Outside limits, though frustrating, are usually a comfort in helping these people know what to expect. By providing some boundaries for Marley, I'd actually gotten our relationship off on the right foot.

The battle had only begun, however. Marley appeared in my office and plopped into a chair. She informed that she had shown up but that I would have to do the talking. I spent a few moments explaining the nature and purpose of our program. Marley listened stonily while I told her I would expect her to talk with me at least three times a week, that she would be participating in group therapy daily, and that she would have to attend lectures and other groups. I finished by asking her to tell me what she would like to get from the program.

She reminded me that all she wanted was to avoid jail. Impatiently, she swung her feet and stared into space, as if waiting for me to dismiss her. I plunged ahead, asking her if she wanted to learn about the mental illness diagnosis she had been given. She told me flatly that the "anger thing" was not *her* problem, but the problem of those who had to be around her. She peered at me intently, as if to gauge my response. I met her gaze, saying nothing. She went on to add that other people just needed to figure out how to treat her and then her "illness" would not be a problem. I asked her how she had felt about my treatment of her on our recent smoke break. Now avoiding my eyes, she said that she had only stayed because she chose to, and that if she had not wanted to stay, she could easily have gotten away from me.

I sensed a facade of bravado that barely covered a hesitancy to her manner that I hadn't seen before. She continued to avoid my gaze as I told her that she seemed strongly invested in keeping people afraid of her. She responded that having people afraid of her was better than nothing. When I asked her if that was what other people gave her—nothing—Marley snapped that she guessed I had not bothered to read her records yet. She said that since she was fourteen years old "they" had been putting her in these places and doing anger management work with her. Bitterly she added that when she tried to calm herself down with marijuana or alcohol, "they" called her an addict.

I waited, hoping Marley would go on, but that appeared to be all the talking she was going to do that day. She consented to listen while I gave her some information about how alcohol and marijuana interfered with her mood stabilizer and also how these substances could increase paranoia, isolation, and her inability to control her impulses and her anger. Her flat affect gave me no indication that she had heard, so we ended the interview shortly after that.

I had stayed past five that day, and the patients were eating their supper when I was called to the patient cafeteria. On my way there, I could hear

Marley screaming all the way down the corridor. In the cafeteria, a nurse and a mental health worker were restraining Marley, who was trying to lunge at another patient and shouting that the patient had taken her food. Loudly, she protested that she'd laid her roll down for a second and the other patient had taken it. The patient Marley spoke of was cowering in her chair, tearful.

With the other staff's help, I steered Marley out into the hallway. I reminded her that the behavior she had just exhibited would not be tolerated. Further, I told her that she was not the only ill person on the unit, and that other highly medicated or detoxing patients might get mixed up about whose food belonged to whom. Marley protested that she still believed the other patient had taken her roll on purpose, but she was calmer and appeared to have gotten the message. I asked her if she could go back and eat her meal without a commotion, and she said she could. As she sauntered back into the cafeteria, her peers eyed her warily, especially the woman she'd accused.

The days passed and, even though we encouraged everyone not to, people mainly treated Marley very carefully, as if she were a bomb due to explode any second. I knew that Marley was used to this kind of treatment, and that it had kept her isolated from any true relationships with others for most of her life. It was time for things to change. The showdown came during Marley's second week in treatment, when Marley and six other patients in my therapy group were talking about marijuana.

Marley, grinning at the group, said she loved marijuana. She boasted that she had grown it, sold it, and smoked it for most of her life. Jamal, who'd just come into treatment and probably hadn't heard about Marley's short fuse, said that he imagined Marley's brain was like a swamp full of THC (tetrahydrocannabinol, the chief intoxicant in marijuana). Then he told her that he did not appreciate her glorifying a drug that was ruining his life. Marley snapped at him to "shut up" and turned her back to him. I observed that Jamal had made a good point about his need not to have the drug glorified and asked what others in the group thought.

The group was wide-eyed and silent, waiting for Jamal or me to be the target for Marley's pent-up rage. Marley stood and swore at me, glaring at me threateningly. Jamal and two other patients stood also, ready to defend me. Firmly, I told Marley she could not stay in the group and act in this manner. I said that if she was going to persist in acting in a threatening way, she would have to leave the group and go to her room.

Marley stood there, and the other patients cringed as we waited to see what she would do. Surprisingly, she said the last thing I'd expected her to say. She protested that this was her group, too, and she belonged here as much as anyone else. I agreed with what she had said but went on to explain that she had to use the group in the way it was supposed to be used, and not to show how different she was from everyone else.

Marley sat down, and so did my three defenders. Jamal turned and grinned at her. He affirmed that this certainly was her group, but that she needed to acknowledge she was not unique. He voiced the truth that the group members were just a bunch of addicts trying to figure out how to get sober. He reminded her that the drug, not the group, was the enemy.

A change came over Marley after that. It was subtle, to be sure, but in saying that she was part of group, she had taken a step toward acting that way. She began to share in limited ways in my group and in others. She opened up to me one-on-one about how excluded she'd always felt and began to acknowledge the ways in which she barricaded herself from others by instilling fear in them. By the time Marley left treatment, she had made an agreement with me that she would stay on her mood stabilizers, she would give sobriety at least a ninety-day shot, and, most of all, she would keep on connecting with people by attending an outpatient program.

In our last meeting, Marley talked about why none of her anger management therapy had ever worked before. She admitted that she had not really cared. She had always believed she was different from everybody else—and probably too ill to get well. She said that here in a dual-diagnosis rehab she had seen people who hear voices, who cut themselves on purpose, and people who could not stop using drugs, even when their lives were being destroyed. She said she guessed maybe she was not the sickest person, after all. Maybe it was time to look at what she did have.

I never saw Marley again after her discharge. I don't know whether her diagnosis was the correct one, or if she might have been scamming us all along. I do know, however, that something in her treatment changed her and that it was a good change. I hope it was enough to put (and keep) her on the road to wellness.

People who may have been thinking of themselves or a family member or friend while reading Marley's story may have wondered which comes first for people—the anger because of isolation, or the isolation because of anger? Clearly, moving away from her strong sense of isolation played an important role in Marley's decision to deal with her misdirected anger.

We may avoid certain people in our lives because of their difficulties with anger. We may be unaware of how many others avoid them as well, and of how long this has been going on, perhaps for many years. What would happen if, instead of avoiding these people, we were to realize that their anger is probably not about us? What would happen if they could begin to experience being a part of something, as Marley did with her group?

Individuals who are in early recovery and are struggling with inappropriate responses to anger can attend twelve-step meetings where they will have the opportunity to share their most upsetting thoughts and feelings—other attendees will still trade phone numbers with them at the end of the meetings. People who have gone through the same scary times in their early recovery can provide experience, strength, and hope, and they will listen and say, "Keep coming back."

Because twelve-step organizations have firm rules governing acting out in these meetings, more often than not, those who attend learn quickly to check their angry or inappropriate responses because they want and need to be a part of a group of people who have been where they are.

Whether a person is angry because of life losses suffered in addiction, post–acute withdrawal, family-of-origin issues, or a chemical imbalance in the brain, that person is still a person. Behind the anger is often hurt, fear, and isolation that keep the person from reaching out to connect with others.

It is important to stress that anger is a productive and healthy response when it is dealt with in healthy ways. An angry response can give us a notion of whether we are safe, vulnerable to mistreatment, or in need of taking action to defend ourselves. People who have been controlled by their anger for much of their lives learn to fear their anger and perhaps other feelings as well. They will profit by learning how to embrace their anger once they know how to direct it.

In the process of learning how not to abuse substances, it is essential that people learn who they are, what they want, and what their role in the world around them is meant to be. For recovering people who are just beginning to let go of their defenses, change comes slowly. The future is not known. Family members, friends, and caregivers can play an important role in helping people in early sobriety to reconnect with the world, to embrace rigorous honesty, and to rebuild the self-respect that they deserve and desire.

WHAT IF I SAY THERE'S MORE THAN ONE ME?

For years, the disorder known as multiple personality disorder has been presented to the public in books and movies, resulting in negative publicity for this disorder. Today this is known as dissociative identity disorder, which is the tendency for a person to show the presence of two or more distinct personalities that recurrently take control of a person's behavior.

Because of the great amount of publicity and public interest surrounding this disorder, some individuals who suffer from mood disorders, episodes of delusion, or mood swings associated with their addiction may believe that they have dissociative identity disorder.

By contrast, families and friends of people whose moods change regularly may overreact to the moodiness without recognizing an underlying disorder. Because of the frequency of false diagnoses, many individuals who actually do have dissociative identity disorder may not receive the attention they require when they speak of their symptoms.

In my years of working in dual-diagnosis rehabilitation, I have seen several individuals who claimed they had more than one personality and were able to name the personalities. This was something that invariably caused chaos in group therapy when individuals would insist that they were different people today than they had been yesterday, and could not remember what had happened in yesterday's group. Counselors often become impatient with these kinds of behaviors, viewing them as the patients' way of being manipulative or of seeking attention. Consequently, individuals who might actually have had this disorder while in our rehab program usually did not stay long, nor did they make much progress.

For people who suffer from addiction, the phenomenon of having two people inside them is not an uncommon one. Most recovering addicts cannot fathom how they can want so badly to stop abusing their substance, yet continue to do so on a daily basis despite immense life losses. They will often refer to the using side of themselves as the "addict inside me" or "my child self." Indeed, addicts have often reported to me how they would weep with regret and disappointment at the same time as they were using, which indicates that both parts of their "selves" were operative. The addict's task in recovery involves learning about this "other self" who sometimes seems to set the addict up to fail. The addict must make an attempt to understand and embrace this "shadow self," as Jung would urge, and finally to understand what it will take for the addict not to win. However, for the addict, this can be done only one day at a time.

When addicts in group therapy are confronted with an individual who may have dissociative identity disorder, they have no sense of the trauma that could have caused a person's identity to split in this way. Also, counselors in dual-diagnosis rehabs (myself included) are usually not schooled in the intensive forms of therapy needed to assist this individual in integrating his or her personalities.

Certainly it is necessary for people who are dually diagnosed to discuss the different ways in which they experience their "selves," but this is often given short shrift by counselors and many caregivers when it spills over into the controversial multiple personality area. As multifaceted individuals, is it not necessary for us to contemplate how diverse we are as we actualize? Do we do a disservice when we steer away from discussions of the complex nature of individuals who, for instance, know they may be delusional at times and may feel as if they are indeed two different people? What about the alcoholic in a black-out who becomes a totally different person, perhaps violent in nature, and the next day remembers none of it? Does this not bear discussing? When faced with the possibility of a person's actually having more than one personality, however, many counselors will avoid discussions about the "parts of oneself," leaving individuals who are seeking wellness with many unanswered questions about why they continue, at times, to react in unpredictable and unfathomable ways.

The vignette that follows presents the story of a person who came to rehab and insisted she had "left her addict at home." Her (and our) dilemma follows.

Arlene's Story

Of all the mental illnesses I have come in contact with as a counselor, dissociative identity disorder has proven to be the most difficult. Oftentimes, clients mistake their mood swings, the voices of their schizophrenia, or their inability to control their impulses for this mental illness, formerly known as multiple personality disorder. Clients may be convinced they have several personalities and treatment becomes focused on their inability to be present to themselves. If the diagnosis truly is dissociative identity disorder (and the client does have more than one personality), it becomes difficult to ascertain whether one is speaking to the personality who is the addict.

Arlene was such a client. An African-American woman of thirty-five, Arlene was friendly and seemingly well-adjusted; she fit in on the unit from the first day. In fact, she had a tendency to be almost *too* cooperative in therapy group, where she tended to assume a cotherapist's role and spent much of the group's time describing her unique mental illness. She warned people in the group that they might see her change at any time. She informed the group that she had at least five or six personalities that she knew of within her. She confided that Jean, the personality who was the cocaine addict, wouldn't come in for treatment. She stated that she was standing in for Jean bodily so that Jean could get back her children who were in custody because of her drug use.

The relish with which Arlene told her story gave me the impression that she was probably making a bid for attention and perhaps exaggerating her symptoms. At any rate, I often had to interrupt her monologues so we could get back to discussing addiction. Still, the group liked to use Arlene to break the boredom, and they'd ask her whether any of her personalities were men or whether they could at least call on Jean and ask to talk to her about her cocaine use.

Arlene stressed in no uncertain terms that the group did not want to meet Jean. She spoke of how mean Jean was, a "real street fighter"—especially when she was craving crack cocaine, as she had been for the past few days. A group member asked Arlene if s*he* was craving cocaine, and, impatiently, Arlene reminded the person that *she* was not the addict, and if it were not for Jean and her antics, she, Arlene, would not even have to be in rehab. So it went, with me struggling to keep the focus off Arlene and on the group process.

One-on-one, Arlene was evasive. She would tell me that she was unable to answer questions about how much cocaine Jean used or what her relapse triggers were. She told me that when Jean took over, she, Arlene, stayed far away. Further, Arlene did not see a need to learn about addiction and I did not have the training or the time to assist her in bringing unity to the disparate parts of her psyche. So we were stuck.

I spent a lot of time, in my discussions with Arlene, talking about what she had lost in her life. She spoke to me about a brutally abusive childhood that she believed had triggered her illness. She told me her mother had been an addict, and, similar to Jean, had liked to fight. She spoke of how people had not been able to reason with her mother. After Arlene's dad left the family, Arlene and her four brothers and sisters were at the mercy of this woman who "went berserk a lot." Arlene described many times when there was no food in the house. She related a story about the time her mother got so angry with her because she had wet herself that she sat her naked on a hot stove burner. Arlene spoke of still having the grim reminder of scar tissue.

As was usually the case when Arlene spoke of her family-of-origin issues, her affect was animated, as if her story was something interesting that had happened to someone else. It was clear she had difficulty experiencing her feelings, those now or in the past. I knew there had to be a volcano of anger within her waiting to be released, if only she could just get in touch with it.

The days went by and Arlene appeared to be one of the most cooperative patients on the unit. One-on-one she was doing little of the work I would usually require a patient to do, and it was never clear to me whether she might be acting in a manipulative fashion to get out of feeling anything. She stopped dominating groups, with my guidance, and did her assignments faithfully. In lectures, she sat up front and took copious notes. In her second week of treatment, she was elected community chairperson and handled the responsibility cheerfully and well. When she was not discussing her personalities, Arlene gave the impression of being someone who didn't even have a mental illness.

Then, one Wednesday afternoon, I was preparing to give a lecture on codependency and Arlene didn't show up. Wondering if she might be sick, I telephoned the nurses' station to ask why Arlene was not in group. "We took her vital signs and there doesn't appear to be anything wrong with her, but she is refusing group," the nurse said. I asked the nurse to send her down and began my lecture.

Five minutes later, an unfamiliar Arlene came slouching into the room. Hair uncombed, clothing disheveled, she appeared to have recently been in bed. She stood just within the doorway glaring at me. When I ignored her and kept on lecturing, she made her way down the aisle, heading toward the back of the room. Her heels hung over the back of her shoes, and every step she took made a loud flapping sound. She took her time, aware that all eyes were on her and not appearing to care. Once settled in the back of the room, she proceeded to put her head down on the desk. I asked Arlene to raise her head, encouraging her to pay attention to the lecture, as she needed to know this material.

When Arlene's head didn't move, I hesitated, trying to figure out what could be wrong with her. I reviewed our morning group, at which she'd been her usual self, and I couldn't recall anything happening that could account for her behavior. Walking to the back of the room, I stood beside Arlene and quietly said her name. Arlene raised her head a fraction and peered at me angrily, mumbling that she did not know who I was talking to, but her name was not Arlene. The room was filled with tension. I imagined many of the patients were recalling, along with me, Jean's tendency to fight. Could this be Jean?

As I moved closer to Arlene's desk, she suddenly stood, violently pushing away the table that was in front of her. She screamed at me to back off as she advanced toward me threateningly. A male patient across the aisle from Arlene jumped up and grabbed her arm, urging Arlene to calm down, promising that no one was going to hurt her. Now Arlene was out of control. She swung blindly at the patient, connecting with his jaw with a loud *thwack*. Without thinking, I stepped between the two of them. Arlene's hand was drawn back to deliver another blow, but seeing me there, she hesitated. Her arm dropped, but rage still flared in her eyes.

By this time the mental health associate was in the room with us. After hitting the panic button to summon more help, she came over to us and put Arlene in the classic restraint position. As other staff came rushing into the room to help, I stood there stunned by how close I had come to putting myself in danger and upset that another patient had been injured because of my lack of vigilance. We all watched Arlene straining and kicking as she was led from the room by three staff members. Her strength was amazing, as was the depth of her anger.

Needless to say, the lecture for the day turned into a session for processing what had just happened. We were shaken by how quickly the turmoil had erupted. All of us had been so certain we knew Arlene. Once the patients were calmer, I ended the group and went to the quiet room where Arlene had been strapped in using four-point restraints. She continued to shout and squirm on the bed where they'd placed her. She said she was not staying in rehab, nor was she going to any more groups. She warned me to get away from her.

We had to spend the next couple of hours waiting for the Youth and Family Services worker who had brought Arlene in to come and pick her up. When we phoned for the pickup, we were careful to warn the worker about Arlene's rage, but she said she knew Arlene would be fine once she was out of the rehab. She said she was almost certain it was Jean we were dealing with, and Jean had been clear about her desire not to be placed in rehab.

I was at a loss and filled with questions. If this worker knew how Jean would respond to finding herself in a rehab, couldn't she at least have warned us? Would Arlene be unable to get her kids back now? Would Jean be high by tomorrow? How would a client on Social Security assistance ever get the intensive therapy she needed to integrate her personalities?

The caseworker promised she would pick up Jean in a couple of hours and apologized for what we'd had to go through with her. Within two hours Arlene was gone from the unit. Nothing remained of her except the small picture of her three kids she'd tacked on my bulletin board one afternoon. She had told me one day that those children were what kept her going. She had also said that it took everything she had to protect the kids from Jean, but she swore that nobody was going to hurt those kids as long as she was around. They were beautiful children, and they appeared well cared for in the picture. What would happen to them now?

Regardless of whether Jean and Arlene actually were two separate personalities, she clearly was incapable presently of being an adequate mother, perhaps even of caring for herself properly. Because the use of addictive substances only complicates a person's mental illness, Arlene would have to remove addictive substances from the picture to integrate her personalities and develop the strength and skills to manage her life.

People who suffer from a fragmented sense of self should seek trained help and proper medication. In the process of receiving counseling, the individual must remain clean and sober, utilizing, whenever possible, a twelve-step group and any other relapse prevention skills he or she may have learned. The Sybils and Eves of books and movies may well have provided us with important examples and information about the nature of personality disorders, but the people who suffer from them still experience much despair and often little support.

We can all identify with the need for self-actualization. For most of us, this is an exciting journey, sometimes painful but not usually devastating. However, the fragmentation created in the lives of people suffering from mental illness and addiction needs to be addressed by trained professionals with the requisite skills and knowledge.

For those of us who are not trained to treat dissociative disorders, but who are only observers of the pain, can we commit to being present to those who may be only partially present to us? Can we make the sacrifice of loving and nurturing those who may not be who they say they are? Can we be there for those who are lost until they can learn, in time, how to be there for themselves?

Chapter 4

The Role of Hope, Empowerment, and Spirituality in Recovery for the Dually Diagnosed Client

An expression in twelve-step programs that describes a person who comes into recovery from addiction and does not relapse is "first-time winner." The ironic point is, I suppose, that one never knows if one truly is a "first-time winner" until the end of one's life. Relapse is always a possibility for the addict, which is why the addict uses the phrase *one day at a time* to describe how long he or she can promise to stay sober. For the dually diagnosed person, the odds of relapse into substance abuse, active mental illness, or both increase.

When patients are compliant on medication, follow their doctors' orders, and still begin to experience symptoms of mental illness, they sometimes give up on sobriety as their judgment becomes impaired.

It is important to understand that, in the battles against addiction and mental illness, each individual's "personal best" varies. Observers of people who relapse continually and cannot hold down a job may say, "Why don't they make an effort?" People who complain that such continual relapses are a financial drain on society may never understand how it feels to be unable, at times, to control one's own actions.

Addiction is an outward reach for inner peace, and many addicts have perhaps not known inner peace for many years of their lives, if ever. As they try to give up their substance abuse and reach inward, they may recall only memories of past failures. They may be convinced that they cannot build inner peace, that they cannot create identities worthy of respect, that they are condemned to failure after failure. The addictive system, which thrives on denial and minimization, often encourages such negative thoughts: "Why even try? You know you can't do it? You'll get sick again and start using. It isn't worth all this effort and pain."

Dually diagnosed individuals who want to learn to stop reaching outside of themselves for pleasure and to cultivate a solid inner core of peace need opportunities to develop hope and spirituality. They need to be empowered to see the strength inside themselves, a strength in which they may have ceased to believe. Many dually diagnosed people who have managed to create this inner core of peace and serenity consider it a miracle. They may say, "My sponsor was able to hope for me when I had lost hope in myself" or "I prayed and my higher power taught me to love myself again."

It is clear that, however this "miracle" occurs, it is not something that people can achieve alone. They need others to connect with, others who will believe in them, give them proper direction, and pick them up when they fall. Twelve-step programs can be strongly directive at times, while still encouraging people to "keep coming back" following relapses and to do "the next right thing."

A dually diagnosed person may not always find answers in twelve-step meetings. The mental illness may prevent the person from feeling comfortable around many unfamiliar people, and the medications and other symptoms may be difficult for other people to understand if they are uninformed about the mental illness. The person may feel alone, unsupported, and misunderstood, and these feelings may contribute to the person's ongoing hopelessness about ever gaining quality of life.

When counselors encourage family members of dually diagnosed persons to show "tough love," this does not mean that they are to give up hope for those people. Indeed, true tough love should convey the message "I know you can do this, and I won't accept anything else except your success. I will detach and let you do what you need to do in order to take care of yourself."

As has been shown in prior chapters, detaching with love is an extremely difficult process. However, if family members want an individual to remain sober and mentally healthy, it is essential that they do not give up hope for this person. Spirituality often comes to a person when he or she feels others have hope and are urging him or her on. The person experiences a sense of being a part of something greater than his or her own inadequate-seeming self. Connected to others, the person feels a new power and sense of self.

Empowerment comes when others offer a role in achieving connectedness. In meetings, people could be given the job of making coffee or the reading aloud of a portion of "the twelve steps." In therapy, people may be given increasing responsibility for the affairs of their lives. With each tiny step forward, they remember what it feels like to succeed and be able to do more.

HOPE

Antonio, whose story is told in the following vignette, remains for me, even now, the embodiment of hope. I feel privileged to have known individuals such as Antonio whose very lives, from one day until the next, hang by the tenuous thread of hope. Antonio's hope was that he would have another day to live and, if not, that he could die simply and with dignity—sober. I still do not know where Antonio found the capacity to hope as he did, spiritually bankrupt as he had become from years of heroin use, but hope he did, and his hope was like a beacon for his peers in treatment, for himself, and for me—even now, years later.

People suffering from addiction can find it very difficult to sustain hope when they first enter treatment. They have come to rely on something outside themselves that they believe can provide all the answers. In so doing, they lose the true answers. Reaching inside themselves, they often find only darkness and despair. It takes time to rebuild an inner core of spirituality that can sustain hope. Newcomers to sobriety often depend on others who can hope for them until they can begin to hope for themselves.

Antonio was dying, but something in his spirit would not die. For him, this hope became the answer to life as he had been meant to live it, just one day at a time.

Antonio's Story

The first time I saw Antonio, I could hardly believe that someone so emaciated could be alive and walking around. I could not help but notice, however, as soon as I met him, the life that shone from his huge brown eyes. He was animated in a way that puzzled me. How could someone who knew he had active AIDS (acquired immunodeficiency syndrome) be so filled with happiness and hope?

An intravenous (IV) heroin user for twenty of his forty years, Antonio had become HIV positive, he believed, ten years ago. His "cocktail" of protease inhibitors had worked for him until about two years ago, when his body had finally given in to a lifetime of abuse and illness. His T cell count had dropped drastically, and in the past winter, he'd been in and out of the hospital numerous times with opportunistic infections.

During our intake I was curious about why Antonio had chosen now, of all times, to get sober. With all the pain and loss of impending death, wouldn't a person want, more than ever, to numb out through addiction? I even wondered to myself if Antonio's frail body would be able to stand the stressors of his recent detox and continuing post–acute withdrawal symptoms.

As we spoke during our first meeting, Antonio's discomfort was obvious. Droplets of perspiration beaded his forehead, and his fingers trembled as he grasped the edge of my desk. He explained to me that, having been a Roman Catholic his entire life, he wanted to come home to God clean and sober. His eyes left mine and glanced downward, as he told me he knew he could get clean from drugs, but he did not know how he could begin to make amends for all the things he had done to get the drugs. He met my gaze again as he asked me if I could assist him in making amends while he was here in rehab.

A stillness settled over the room that sometimes comes during counseling sessions that to me means I am in the presence of complete honesty and a desire for change. I told Antonio that I would like to help him with what he was asking. I added that a person's desire and intention to make amends are the most important parts of the process.

In the days ahead, as I got to know Antonio better, I heard the story of his childhood in a Spanish neighborhood of New York City. He'd been the child of a prostitute and, as her oldest son, had assumed the task of looking out for his mother and his four younger siblings. He'd been a gang member and had dabbled in street drugs since the age of nine. Long before he began shooting heroin he'd been no stranger to crime. He told me that he and his friends had done what they had to do to survive. He had not felt it was such a bad thing to steal, he said, when his brothers and sisters were hungry. Antonio also said that he'd been in and out of the church as a youngster, and he spoke of those experiences with a reverence that showed that the church had been a touchstone for him. He would go into the church to light a candle, though he admitted that he did not know why. Maybe, he said, it was a kind of prayer—a prayer he hoped someone somewhere would hear.

By the time Antonio was thirteen, his mother had disappeared. After his siblings were taken into foster care and he lost touch with them, for seven years, he had lived on the street, supporting himself in a number of ways, including male prostitution. Antonio admitted he was gay and also that he never had been sure whether he had become HIV positive through unprotected sex or because of a dirty needle. He became tearful as he spoke to me about his life as a gay man. He sobbed as he told me he did not want God to judge him for his lifestyle. He wondered if God had seen and knew of his struggles—a small child who had seen men doing things to his mother that he would never do to anyone. He went on to say that he had never really found a love that felt right to him, and he was frightened that, when he died in a few weeks, no one would be there for him. He hoped that his making amends spiritually would change this.

In the days that followed, Antonio's social worker began putting together a support system for him within the HIV-positive organizations that are available in our state. Antonio had already been going to support meetings and had been scheduled to move into housing for individuals with full-blown AIDS. The one thing we could not put into place for him, however, was a family—someone who would see him through until the end. Ironically, this was not necessarily due just to his poor lifestyle choices, to his drug use, or to his criminal activities. Antonio had never really known a family and he was realizing now, in this vulnerable time, how much he had missed.

We spoke of twelve-step groups, a sponsor, and a home group. As I watched Antonio in the milieu of our rehab, I was touched by how the other patients reached out to him as if he were the strong one. Frail as he was physically, he did have a strength of spirit that others recognized. I knew, watching him interact in treatment, that he would be accepted in this same way in the rooms of AA and NA.

Antonio began to attend twelve-step meetings in our rehab program. Often, people who come into our facility to run twelve-step meetings will volunteer to act as a patient's sponsor when they come out of rehab. Antonio found such a person in the second week of his treatment, and I let him use my phone daily to touch base with the man. At the end of one such conversation, Antonio told me the man had agreed to pick him up and take him to twelve-step meetings after his discharge. Antonio had been wondering for a long time how he would get to meetings, with no transportation available to him, and he saw this as an answer to his prayer.

I couldn't believe I was counseling a patient who was grateful for such a small thing. Often, patients view meetings as a job or an inconvenience. Here was a man who knew he could not save his life, yet he wanted to attend daily meetings. Antonio was focused on saving his soul—and perhaps that was the difference.

Since the first day I had met Antonio, I had wondered why he had been referred to our dual-diagnosis unit, because I was not sure I saw evidence of mental illness. As time went on, though, I began to see in him the dementia the doctors had mentioned in his diagnosis. Many people with full-blown AIDS show evidence of brain involvement from the disease that manifests itself in depression, forgetfulness, paranoia, and, sometimes, unexplainable anger.

At times, Antonio would forget what we had talked about in a previous session. Periodically, an unnatural quietness would come over him, and he would not want to talk to me. I had difficulty determining whether these were the natural behaviors of someone who knew he had a limited amount of time to live, or whether they were part of the dementia. It was clear to me, though, that Antonio was holding on to his mind with all that he was worth. With his mind, his very spirit, he was struggling to keep intact, and I felt immense respect for that. My counseling consisted mainly of listening to a litany of "getting honest." At the end of each item he related, Antonio expressed his remorse for what he had done and for whom he had hurt. I wondered how it must feel to be a priest and wished I had the power to grant absolution to this remarkable person sitting in front of me.

Too soon, Antonio's twenty-one days were completed. On the last day, as we sat in the small-group meeting and each person said a few words while holding the medallion Antonio would receive as a token of program completion, many tears fell. We all knew we would not see him again. At the end of the group, as I was the last person to pass the medallion, I stood and hugged Antonio. I could feel his bony shoulders beneath his shirt and the fine tremor that never seemed to leave him, but I also felt a surge of spiritual strength within this man, who'd come to us to do a difficult thing and had succeeded. "You earned this," I whispered, pressing the medallion into his hand. Holding the medallion aloft, Antonio said that he knew the medallion was a sign that he had gotten what he came for—a home for his spirit. For Antionio, the medallion symbolized much more than sobriety.

Antonio left that afternoon, but he remained in my thoughts. Now and then I would hear from someone who had seen him at a meeting, and I knew that he was continuing to follow his program. In the spring, four months down the road, just as the leaves were budding, I heard that Antonio had died. Our unit clerk received a phone call from Antonio's sponsor. He wanted us to know that Antonio had died clean and sober, and, the sponsor affirmed, he had been at peace.

Individuals such as Anthony bring into rehab a positive energy that is healing to all of us. His hope that he could change not only his actions but the very essence of his spirit infected us all. Individuals such as Antonio live out the miracle of the twelve-step saying about believing in a power greater than ourselves to help restore us to sanity. For Antonio, what began as the tiny bit of hope he could muster to light a candle was passed on to an entire recovery community, this counselor included, and then grew to the size of a bonfire.

EMPOWERMENT

The most difficult part of helping an individual become empowered, I have found, is needing to remain firm in not doing for that individual what I know he or she can do unassisted. However, if this individual appears greatly impaired, do I not take a risk in perhaps requiring too much of the person? Further, if this individual has been benefiting from a lifetime of having others fulfill his or her needs, how can I assure this person that more will be gained by being self-sufficient?

The process of empowerment is in no way an exact science. Empowering people requires an intuitive sense of who they are, what they can do, and what desires (perhaps unknown to them) propel them forward in life. Those who have this kind of intuitive sense are naturally more focused on others' welfare than on their judgments of others. Empowering people to accomplish their own life tasks requires risk and self-sacrificing, since people are often not happy with those who nudge them forward, no matter how gentle that nudging might be.

Many times I have required behaviors or progress from individuals when I have not been sure that they could or would rise to the occasion. I have learned, though, that individuals who are unable to meet expectations in an empowering situation may still appreciate the respect they have been shown simply because something was expected of them. Other individuals who were also motivated by my expectations of them appeared to learn as much from the experience of making an effort on their own behalf as they did by reaching the goal.

I have found that, when empowering someone, I don't always know what the definition of success in each instance will be. Probably the real success comes in the person's accepting the challenge of moving toward self-sufficiency and all the risks and losses that may imply. Individuals who wish to be empowered must, as a first step, stop underestimating themselves. Often, individuals with mental illness or addiction have no real sense of their capabilities. Their addictive thinking and/or mental state may have dictated, for years, everything they believed they could not do. Many people in early recovery are terrified of failure, and even more may be afraid of success. To forge forward alone when neediness and perceived inability to succeed provide a comfortable place to hide is courageous. However, as I have seen numerous times, the human spirit requires more of us than the acceptance of a hiding place throughout life. Only by risking and moving into the unknown can people discover their abilities and, most important, develop self-respect along the way.

Individuals who seek to empower others must be willing to risk being resisted and disliked strongly—perhaps for quite some time. Most people, especially those with disabilities, resist change at the outset. They do not easily see, in the beginning, the respect implied when demands are made of them. Only in retrospect, after progress has been made, will what was achieved by the empowering process become apparent. Even if it never becomes apparent, it is necessary to care about the people one wishes to empower, without the promise of thanks. That is a tall order for many of us.

As a counselor, I have learned that a patient's anger directed toward me usually means I'm doing something right. Empowering the people with whom I have worked has been one of the most difficult skills I have had to embrace as a counselor. Working with dually diagnosed people who may have struggled for years to address the simplest tasks of life, I have reacted too many times with inappropriately strong sympathy or an immediate desire to make the person more comfortable. Only after long experience have I learned that the pain I see in patients is, most likely, something they need to feel before seeking change. Thus, the alcoholic's question to another alcoholic—"Have you reached your bottom yet?"—begins to make sense. The people I saw in rehab were usually at a point in their lives where their pain had gotten their attention. For me to alleviate that pain (instead of teaching them how to do it) might take away their one opportunity to see where they were at and address the condition of their lives. Watching individuals struggle through their pain and move forward, seeing them change and grow is enough for me to know that I am not being cruel or uncaring when I don't offer a hand someone may not need.

The vignette that follows presents an individual who required strong limits before beginning to move forward. Susan, wounded from years of abusive treatment, could not stand people looking at her. Hidden behind dark glasses, she lived in her own world and did not want to come out. Susan illustrates the great hostility that is often displayed by a person who wants to be left alone in that safe niche of isolation. Her facade of confidence and imagined self-sufficiency were daunting, to say the least, but even more daunting was the process of trying to see behind that facade and to help Susan set it aside.

Susan's Story

Because of her "funky" appearance, Susan almost didn't make it onto our dual-diagnosis unit. It was not that she didn't meet our dress code; she had thought of infringements to a dress code we didn't even have. Completely enveloped in man-sized overalls over a baggy psychedelic blouse, her body was an unknown quantity. Was she fat, slim, in-between? Who knew? To top that off, she wore heavy combat-style boots into which she'd tucked the bottoms of her overalls. To complete the unbroken shield behind which she hid, her hair swirled around her head in a bouffant blonde mop, ending beyond the rim of the huge sunglasses with which she covered her eyes. Dangling from the blonde mop was a cascade of multicolored paper clips that she had fashioned into an earring; the top paper clip was hooked into her pierced ear.

A driver had left Susan and her patient records at the nurses' station and had quickly left the premises. We had no one to consult about Susan's appropriateness for our program. The head nurse approached Susan (squaring her shoulders, as she always did when having to set limits at the outset). She firmly told Susan to hand over the glasses, as they were forbidden on the unit.

Susan backed away. She muttered from beneath her hair that she needed the glasses for medical reasons. I noticed that Susan kept pursing her lips. I thought that she could be nervous or maybe she had tardive dyskinesia, a side effect of psychotropic medications. In either case, it was clear she was all set to stand fast.

When clients come to our unit, they are seen on admission by our psychiatrist as soon as possible. In Susan's case, this was very soon. We were certain that she would be found inappropriate for the unit, allowing us to move on with our day. Not so. Within an hour, I found out that the doctor had managed to confiscate Susan's paper clip earring, but the rest of Susan's getup was going to remain. The doctor informed the treatment team that Susan had a sensitivity to light and did need the dark glasses. He stated he had encouraged Susan to remove the glasses when she was in a room that was sufficiently dark for her not to have a reaction, but otherwise she would be wearing them on the unit and outside at smoke break.

Before I met with Susan that afternoon for an intake, I spent a lot of time reading the patient information chart that had been sent to us from her aftercare program, and it explained a lot. Susan's mother had been an active heroin user for most of Susan's life. Her father had been unknown—just one of many men Susan's mother slept with to pay for her habit. Susan had been raised mostly by her grandmother, a well-meaning woman, according to reports, but inattentive and routinely unable to deal with Susan's acting-out behaviors.

The acting-out behaviors included Susan's cutting herself regularly from the age of eight, bingeing and purging from the age of thirteen, promiscuity (resulting in two children whom the grandmother took in), and drug abuse (crack, heroin, PCP, ecstasy, methamphetamines, and marijuana). Susan had come to us because her grandmother wanted her out of the house and permanent custody of Susan's kids, a boy (age three), and a girl (age seven). By receiving treatment, Susan was hoping she might stand a chance of keeping custody of her children.

Reading about Susan's history of self-mutilation, I wondered if she'd had a history of sexual abuse or some other form of severe childhood trauma, which often leads to incidents of self-mutilation. Susan's program had given her a diagnosis of borderline personality disorder, a mental illness that manifests itself by a person's having ongoing difficulty establishing or maintaining intimacy with others because of boundaries broken in early childhood. Self-mutilation, eating disorders, and substance abuse are often the person's ways of comforting the self and of awakening long-suppressed feelings.

So I knew that Susan was going to be a tough case. If I did manage to win her trust, at some point she would push me away, I knew, because too much closeness can feel threatening to someone with borderline personality disorder. "Set limits," I'd always been taught. "People with this disorder need limits."

An hour later Susan sat, or rather slouched, in the chair across from me. It was disconcerting not being able to see her eyes. Her papers had said she was twenty-five years old, but she looked even younger sitting there. Still, as invisible as Susan was to me physically, I could definitely feel the strength of her personality, an aura emanating from her. I decided to be silent and see what she'd do. Finally, she asked me to explain why she was in the place and what was expected of her. I countered by asking her why she thought she was here. Susan sat silently pursing her lips. Maybe, even, she was forcing back a smile. Susan said she guessed I wanted to check her out and fix her, as had the rest of the people who'd been "shrinking" her for all these years. She crossed one booted foot over her knee and told me to "go to it."

I wondered aloud what Susan thought needed fixing. Grinning, she told me she really would be fine if the drugs didn't keep running out. She said it was times such as these, when she had to sit in front of someone—anyone—clean and sober, that she felt like "freaking out." She continued by saying that she had been born on drugs, since her mother had used heroin during her pregnancy. With studied indifference, she added that her mom had died a couple of years before. I was silent, thinking of all the people I'd counseled who'd become addicted to drugs while they were in their mothers' wombs. Some never seemed to get past it. I wondered, once again, what it must it be like to come into the world addicted and to have to go through withdrawal at birth.

Susan continued, describing the men who had come into her mother's apartment and the sexual things they had done to Susan when she was no more than a toddler. She finished by giving me an intent look and asking me if that was what I had wanted to hear. I stayed silent. Though I wanted to reach out and offer some kind of comfort, I knew this would feel too intimate for Susan, especially as she was recalling the invasion of her boundaries. So I listened as years of pain poured out of Susan's memory. At one point, I leaned forward and flicked off my office light. Slowly, Susan removed her glasses, and I could see tears welling in her eyes.

Now and then, as we talked, the glasses went back on, as if what she had revealed was too much. Sometimes, when she took the glasses off, she would also sweep the blonde mop off her forehead, and I could see that she was truly beautiful—but not, I was sure, to herself.

That was the beginning of a healing time for Susan, but it didn't come without her resisting me all the way. At the end of our session, Susan put her fighting gear (and attitude) back on and went out into the unit to tell the staff what she would and would not tolerate. Also, the next time she saw me in the hall, she turned her head and did not speak.

Approach and retreat is a classic coping mechanism for individuals with borderline personality disorder, and therapists, friends, and family would do well to remember that and not take the behavior personally. Susan acted out in my therapy group, she often did not show up for appointments, and she clung like crazy to her oversized clothing and her dark glasses. Through all of this I did set limits, realizing that Susan had not had limits set for her previously in her life. I told her I expected to see her (on time) when we made an appointment, and if she was not on time she would lose the appointment. Further, I told her that if she was inappropriate in group, she would be asked to leave until she felt more in control.

Confrontations such as these would always be followed by a good session with Susan, often with her glasses removed. I remained consistent with her, and she began to appear to know what to expect. She seemed to understand that my consistency was my way of showing I cared and that, sometimes, she could expect it from other healthy people around her as well.

The twenty-one days she spent in our rehab program went by quickly. Susan became friends with some of the young nurses on the evening shift and began to open up to them too. One of the nurses spoke to Susan about her lovely skin and features, encouraging Susan to wear a headband to sweep her hair off her forehead. Some of Susan's female peers loaned her normal-sized jeans and sweatshirts, and I came in one day to a practically unrecognizable Susan—hair pulled back from her face and normal young person's attire. We were making progress. Of course, the dark glasses were still mostly ever present.

Up until the last week, Susan had never really opened up in group therapy. Three days before her discharge, we were talking in group therapy about children. Almost everyone in the group had kids and several were there to regain custody of those kids. Susan burst out at one point, interrupting the person who was talking, to ask how she could possibly keep her kids from going what she went through if the system took them away from her. I reminded Susan that good parents do not use illegal drugs, they do not use in front of their children, and they are not emotionally unavailable to them.

Susan countered that she was certainly aware of what I was saying, but she didn't know how she could be any kind of parent feeling as awful as she did all the time. She began to sob and pulled her glasses off to wipe her eyes, saying that, without drugs, life felt unbearable to her. One of her peers got up and quietly shut off the lights in the room and brought Susan a tissue. Another of her peers leaned toward Susan and confided that he, too, felt horrible without drugs. He went on to say that he knew, though, that the feelings would pass in time. He assured her that, as much as he had already seen Susan change, he thought she could stay clean until she started feeling better. The group murmured its agreement.

The lights stayed off. Susan's glasses stayed off. For the rest of the time in group therapy that day, we spoke about what feeling normal is. Sometimes it *is* feeling awful, and that's when we can begin to address the issues in our lives that make us feel that way. Susan received her recovery medallion three days later in the group. Everyone there knew she had earned it. Glasses off, face shining, she told us that she was going to try "to be normal."

Susan had reluctantly come out from behind her self-imposed barricade to connect and, in that, she had been nurtured. I don't have the good fortune of hearing from many of my patients after they leave rehab. Sometimes I see them when they come back through following a relapse. Susan? I'd like to think that she made it out there—that she is showing her face and her beautiful spirit to the world as she showed them to us in our treatment center.

From Susan's story, it is possible to see the incremental nature of the empowerment process. Gradually, but continuously, she was prodded to come out of hiding, first physically with her hair, clothing, and glasses, and, finally, emotionally. Susan had not been accustomed to feeling validated by others. When the other people in her group therapy sessions validated her feelings by acknowledging them and admitting that they shared many of her feelings, she perhaps began to see her journey forward as not so solitary. It is interesting to note that the main source of empowerment for Susan while in rehab was her peers, suggesting that the intuitiveness necessary to empower someone does not reside in only trained counselors or people who are sober for many years.

SPIRITUALITY

The concept of spirituality has long been central in twelve-step recovery circles. It is, in fact, the basis of the "miracle" that allows people who are addicted to refrain, one day at a time, from engaging in an obsession that has been destroying them. People who seek recovery from addiction often, in the beginning, confuse the concept of spirituality with religion. When they conceive of surrendering their will and their lives to a higher power (of their understanding), they often feel as if they are being preached to or that they are being asked to accept the tenets of a religion. What is really being stressed, however, is the notion that individuals who wish to stop being ruled by their obsessions must, first of all, accept that they have an obsession (addiction) and that they are powerless over it. Once they are in this place emotionally, they must then come to believe that some force or power *can* help them, since they have seen countless other powerless individuals deal with their obsessions in this mysterious way and remain clean and sober.

Thus begins the process of acceptance and surrender. Individuals begin, in seeking spirituality, to explore ways of putting aside their self-will. They begin to consider what might happen in their lives if they start to believe that a power greater than themselves is willing to assist them. They begin to align themselves with this power in the hopes that self-destructive patterns may change, one day at a time.

For addicts, the habit of feeding their unappeasable hunger for substances now becomes a process of self-emptying. A giant leap of faith is required of people who have so avidly reached outside themselves to fill this hunger—perhaps for a lifetime—now just to stop and wait. The unappeasable hunger is still there, but they now know that what they have reached for did not feed them but instead caused them to feel empty inside—a spiritual void. Filling that particular void, in many cases, involves finding a higher power.

The process of finding spirituality—or of contacting one's own spirit and of learning how to connect with the spirit in others—is the very basis of the kind of wellness discussed in the preceding chapters. Whether people have a recurring mental illness that impacts their lives, whether they are addicts who happen to be mentally ill as well, or whether they struggle with the inner void that all of us experience at times in our lives, spirituality is integral to their actualization and to their knowledge of themselves as beings who matter in the world. How each individual finds a way to be spiritual is a private matter.

For people who are dually diagnosed and for their families, twelve-step programs can be of immense help, as they teach, through their practices and principles, ways of living in the moment, ways of accepting what is, and ways in which people may affirm themselves and take responsibility for their actions—thus creating self-respect and a nurturing spirit.

In my work with dually diagnosed people, I have been called on time and again to define what is meant by spirituality. Addicts, so accustomed to acquiring what they need immediately, think of it as something they need to "get"—and the sooner the better. I tell people that spirituality is more something that one has to "allow." By emptying oneself, by stopping self-seeking, by being willing to acknowledge that others are willing to help if one would wait and let that help take the form it is supposed to take—one makes the first faltering step toward an understanding of spirituality. It is then that the miracle can begin to happen.

Sometimes the greater the suffering, the higher the level of spirituality. Perhaps the need for a higher power becomes greatest when individuals have no other choice but to surrender on a daily basis. Fred, whose story is told in the following vignette, was an example of people I have known who seemed to walk around with a childlike faith that the rest of us were always struggling to understand and achieve for ourselves. Fred often exemplified, far better than any teaching I could do, what spirituality could mean in a person's life.

Fred's Story

"This guy won't do much here" was my first thought when I saw Fred ambling down the hall, his eyes averted and his shaved head gleaming. A cross between cool and disheveled, Fred was hard to pin down. Clearly, he was one of the homeless guys who had come to our inpatient dual-diagnosis rehab for twenty-one days' worth of "hots and a cot." Fred had come in over a weekend and I hadn't gotten to do an intake with him, so my impression of him remained negative as he sat in our first group therapy session, his elbows on his knees and his head down. Staring at his feet, he seemed to have little interest in anything anyone was saying.

When I called on him to share, he looked up at me, startled, as if he'd been somewhere else. He murmured that he did not have much to say. He did know that drinking was the only thing that made his "voices" go away, and for that reason, he had been drinking for thirty years. He admitted he'd gotten into crack cocaine the past few years, but that made his voices worse and they sometimes said some "not so nice" things. His head dropped down again and the group was silent, processing what he'd shared.

A female in the group asked Fred if he took his medication on a regular basis. She said that her medication made her voices go away most of the time, unless she was under stress. Fred, without raising his head, admitted that it was hard for him to figure out how to get his medication and when to take it. He shrugged, clearly eager for us to move on to someone else.

After group, I wrote Fred's name on my appointment chalkboard on the door of my office and waited for him to show up at two o'clock. Two o'clock came and went with no Fred. Later that afternoon, as the clients were lining up to be taken out for smoke break, I went to see Fred to ask him why he hadn't kept his appointment. He told me he did not know of any appointment. His eyes were on the line of those going out to smoke, and I could see he was eager to join them. I reminded Fred that I was his counselor and that I had told him in therapy group that we would be doing an intake together at two o'clock. Fred repeated that he did not know about that. He held up his hands and studied his fingers. For the first time, I noticed how ashy the skin was on his hands, the knuckles worn and creased, skin flaking and dry. He asked me, in a low voice, when I wanted to talk. When he finally did look at me, I saw fear and confusion. It occurred to me that Fred probably had brain damage in addition to his schizophrenia. What had originally appeared to be street cool and attitude had been Fred's way of trying to fit in. I told Fred we would talk when he came back from smoke break. I turned and pointed to my office door. "In here, Fred. Soon as you come up."

Fifteen minutes later Fred was at my door. He asked if this was when we were supposed to talk, as he shifted from one foot to the other. Smiling to reassure him, I invited him in. Pulling out the sheet of questions I usually ask on intake, I put it aside. I knew that Fred wouldn't take well to my writing down what he said. The next forty-five minutes were a revelation. Fred began his long history of not remembering at the age of five when he had fallen (or may have been pushed) out a second-floor window. He told the story with little affect, as if it had been a perfectly normal incident. He said there had been twelve children in his family, and he knew it had been difficult for his parents to keep up with them all. He'd been taken to a neighbor's after the fall, not to a hospital.

Fred's account of his life was sketchy. He had begun hearing voices that commanded him to do things by the age of sixteen and had started drinking shortly afterward to make the voices go away. Since then he'd had nearly a dozen psychiatric hospitalizations (he thought), and each time he had come out sicker, more confused, and with more life losses.

Most amazing, though, was the way Fred began to open up to me once I had won his trust. When I asked him what his dream for his life had always been, he looked right at me and smiled as he said that he had always wanted to be a preacher, to preach about the goodness of God because God had been so very good to him. I asked him to go on, fascinated at Fred's take on a life that had sounded desolate and filled with misery.

Fred said that he was reassured, on a daily basis, by his higher power that things were going to be okay. He spoke of all the people who had been sent to help him in his life. He grinned as he talked about a shelter he went to on a regular basis, where he was allowed to work in the thrift shop. He said the food was good and the counselors there had helped him to get a room of his own. He said his one wish was to go back there once he was able to get off the crack cocaine. People on the street liked him, he admitted, and they just kept giving cocaine to him. Shaking his head, he said he knew he needed to learn how to say "no."

I could see why people liked Fred. Glancing down at the blank intake form in front of me, I realized that this time with Fred had not seemed like work. Where could I start with a guy who had more humility and gratitude than I ever would? Most of his memory problems were short term, as is often the case with the end-stage alcoholic. I found during the next three weeks that making appointments just didn't work for Fred. Several times a day he would appear at my door, wanting to talk. I wasn't sure how I could teach Fred much about refusal skills and relapse prevention. More than once, in our talks, I wondered if Fred might not be there to teach me.

Fred attended groups with the help of his peers, who herded him to the right rooms at the right times. In group he would sit, eyes fastened on his feet, as was customary. I knew now, however, that he was listening, despite how he looked, and, sometimes, he gave the most amazing feedback. When one time we were discussing abandonment issues, a female in the group sobbed that her mother had never cared about her and nothing she ever did was enough, Fred, staring at his feet, quietly asked her if she had ever thought how it had been for her mother. He suggested that she might not know how her mother really felt about her because, sometimes, people act differently than they feel.

The woman stared at Fred speculatively, agreeing that her mom had not had an easy time of it. She recalled that her mom's father had "messed with her" sexually when she was a child and wondered whether he had done that to her mom when she was small as well. She rubbed her eyes, calmer, focused now on her mom rather than herself. Others in the group began to chime in, sharing things that they'd just begun to realize about why their own parents had treated them the way they had. Fred was silent, but still listening.

It got to the point where I began to look for Fred between groups. I looked forward to our brief talks. I took sustenance from his simple acceptance of life and his lot. I did my job with him, role-playing how he'd turn down crack cocaine the next time it was offered to him and talking about NA and AA meetings. Mostly, however, I listened to him, knowing that whatever Fred didn't have was not as important as what he did have. He had made, in the midst of severe and persistent mental illness, the connection. He'd made it with others and with his higher power.

Would it keep him sober? Would it keep him alive? That I do not know. On his discharge day, as I gave him his twenty-one-day medallion, I told him that, of all the clients I had worked with in a long time, I would miss him the most. And I have.

In this discussion of hope, empowerment, and spirituality, I have been emphasizing, most of all, each person's need for dignity. Helping a person get well and stay well requires acknowledging, at all times, that person's need for dignity. The ravages of addiction and active mental illness can make severe inroads on people's ability to access their dignity. They may need someone else to hope for them and to gently prod them toward affirming their wavering faith in themselves. They may need someone who has lived "many days at a time" in surrender to model for them what it is to have faith that a higher power can and will help. Down the road, after many years' worth of "days at a time," these people may themselves need someone else to whom they can reach out so that, in that connection, they recall, with gratitude and humility, where they have been.

Chapter 5

What the Consumer and the Family of the Consumer Can Do Today to Improve Treatment Options

When I give lectures to the dually diagnosed clients I counsel, I say to them, "You are the most courageous people I know." They usually stare at me in disbelief when I say this. They are not used to praise or approval. Many of them believe, as a lot of people do, that courage is about achieving a lot, owning a lot, and having strong self-esteem. They think, too, that courageous people do not fall ill over and over again. They do not go out and use illegal drugs, even if it is to self-medicate, and, most of all, they do not hurt their families by doing the same stupid things over and over again.

For people with a dual diagnosis, wellness is often defined as short periods of stability sandwiched between multiple relapses. In fact, dually diagnosed individuals I have worked with have sometimes become suicidal in the face of their continuing inability to remain stable for long periods of time.

Yet, as you have seen in the vignettes of previous chapters, these are people who pull themselves out of chaos again and again. They are people who, despite their pain, are able to reach out to others and have compassion for them. Eleanor, who feared she'd be mugged in treatment, found a loving family who helped her to reembrace living. Fred, who could barely remember where his room was because of his brain impairment, gave feedback in groups that helped other people get well. Antonio, who was dying, wanted to give up heroin and make amends.

It's true that addicts are manipulative and often dishonest people—able to con their families and society as a whole. These very characteristics, a part of the disease that is addiction, however, also cause addicts to become isolated. Lost within themselves and their addic-

tions, they find themselves in a downward spiral. Until dually diagnosed individuals are able to be guided out of this morass of dis-
connectedness and hopelessness, they are doomed. Getting them to
want this guidance is the first step in providing treatment.

Dually diagnosed individuals, their families, friends, and clinicians encounter great obstacles to treatment at every turn. Susan, born
of a heroin-addicted mother, was impaired in ways many of us will
never be able to understand. Candy, able to get over-the-counter
ephedra to maintain her anorexic lifestyle, became psychotic as a result. Then there was Jesús, whose mother kept him at home so she
could benefit from his check but had him arrested for drinking the
beer that she kept in the house. Some dually diagnosed individuals
have been scapegoated in their families, as Allan was; some are so
good at scamming, as Josh was, that they never receive any help,
though they desperately want to live; and others, such as Melanie, see
themselves as sexual objects.

No therapist can make a new scenario for the dually diagnosed client that is free of abuse, enablement, misunderstanding, disrespect,
and neglect. What therapists, families, and friends of the dually diagnosed person can do, however, is to understand and address the many
ways that can make his or her passage through the world less circu-
itous and self-defeating.

I have treated many dually diagnosed individuals who were unable
to get Supplemental Security Income even though they were severely
disabled by their mental illness. Without a check or medical coverage, they were forced to try to work (and often fail) or commit crimes
(and be arrested or hospitalized). For some, this went on for years until they no longer had the credibility to receive services and were
known as people who had "burned all their bridges."

I have seen families who welcome their family members home
from rehab by throwing a large party, with booze, and later complain,
when the clients go to AA meetings, that they are never home and
must be drinking. These same families complain when the dually diagnosed individuals want to go to an outpatient program for a few
weeks until they have had at least ninety days sober, thinking they
should be working and not hanging around with other addicts.

Some families and program workers make promises to clients, if
they'll just agree to go to rehab but then don't fulfill those promises
later. Some clients come to rehab and do well, but their family mem-

bers do not call or visit and later sever all ties. Program workers, too, are notorious for calling us while clients are in rehab to tell us the clients cannot come back to that program, even though they sent the clients to us with the promise that they could come back after the twenty-one days.

How does one maintain hope in the face of so many inconsistencies? Thankfully, in my years of doing this work, I have seen people bounce back more often than not. The resiliency some dually diagnosed individuals possess is reflected in the stories you have just read. For people such as those portrayed in the vignettes, treatment options can be improved in various ways.

Beyond addressing the problems of family dysfunction, treatment resistance issues, and misunderstandings about dual diagnosis, counselors, families, and friends need to advocate for improved treatment options for individuals who are dually diagnosed. This cannot begin to happen until there is a greater understanding of the needs of the dually diagnosed client and how they may best be met. It is clear that the issues of addiction and mental illness need to be understood more and feared less within families and society.

GETTING WELL: FINDING AND RECEIVING APPROPRIATE DUAL-DIAGNOSIS TREATMENT

Change and progress in the treatment of dually diagnosed people will occur only with an effective continuum of care. The following list presents clear-cut ways, if you are a dually diagnosed individual or the family member or friend of a dually diagnosed individual, to find and receive effective treatment:

1. Recognize and identify the problem. Individuals who believe they may have a substance abuse problem need to be assessed by a trained addiction counselor. Sometimes a family intervention may be necessary before individuals recognize the need to be assessed. Individuals who believe they have a mental illness need to seek a referral from their primary care doctor for a psychiatrist who can perform a psychiatric evaluation. The psychiatrist can provide insight into whether medication or hospitalization will be necessary and discuss treatment options. It is

essential that family members come to the psychiatrist with the individuals to offer caring, tactful input about symptoms.

2. Once problems are identified, and the individuals are ready to address them, it is helpful to receive referrals to appropriate treatment facilities and levels of care from the psychiatrist, social worker, or case manager who has been working with the family.

3. Once it is established which treatment facilities are within traveling distance and are accepted by the individuals' insurance plans, family members should visit these facilities to ask questions about the daily schedule and the availability of an on-site psychiatrist and to acquaint themselves with the rules and guiding principles of the facility. Dually diagnosed individuals should be treated in a facility that provides a combined dual-diagnosis approach, if possible.

4. It is important to establish whether the dually diagnosed individuals will need to undergo detoxification from their substance before attending an outpatient program. Alcoholics who have been drinking for many years can be at risk for seizure if they are not detoxified gradually from alcohol. Crisis units in local hospitals can do withdrawal assessments and determine whether detoxification is necessary.

5. Once the individuals are receiving outpatient care for addiction, they will learn how to find AA and/or NA meetings and how to use them. Most outpatient programs will require that dually diagnosed individuals find a sponsor (a person with several years' sobriety) to help them locate meetings and secure transport to them, and generally to manage their sobriety.

6. Outpatient programs can assist dually diagnosed individuals in finding places to live within the community once they have established some sobriety and are stable on medications. Group homes, Oxford Houses (groups of recovering men and women who rent homes together), and residential programs will be recommended to families when the time is right. Again, it is essential that families and dually diagnosed individuals visit these places to ensure that they will be appropriate. Often, these are halfway or three-quarter houses that individuals will need only in the beginning, until they are well enough to live on their own.

7. Ongoing therapy for family members and for the dually diagnosed individuals may be necessary. When relapses occur, when addicts experience stress, when medications don't work, they need to have access to someone who is trained and available for consultation.

8. Most important, consumer advocacy must be undertaken by dually diagnosed individuals and their families. Once dual diagnosis is fully understood by the people who live with it, they should educate those who may not fully understand.

ENSURING WELLNESS FOR ALL: THE NEED FOR ADVOCACY FOR IMPROVED DUAL-DIAGNOSIS TREATMENT

The Counsel for Substance Abuse Treatment (CSAT) published a recent Treatment Improvement Protocol (TIP #9) that strongly emphasizes the need for combining substance abuse and mental illness treatment, a protocol that should be one of the strongest foci of advocacy groups in all states. The counsel strongly recommends that dually diagnosed individuals and their families become knowledgeable about federal grant monies available to support treatment. The counsel also recommends that dually diagnosed people and their families be offered roles in the training process for dual-diagnosis staff, be included on advisory boards for nonprofit and government treatment programs, and be offered the opportunity to train as peer counselors.

Often, dually diagnosed people may seek treatment from their primary health providers who may have insufficient training about mental health and addiction. Mentally ill people who need medication might be denied it if the doctors view the patients' addiction as the main problem and urge abstinence as a primary goal. When dually diagnosed individuals do not have available to them the combined resources of mental health and addiction professionals working together, the best treatment cannot be provided.

As we seek to provide more comprehensive and focused dual-diagnosis treatment, who would know better what their needs are than dually diagnosed individuals themselves? The most effective conferences I have attended have been those which have included consumers as speakers and members of panels receiving questions from myself and my peers. In cases such as these, provision of treatment transcends theoretical notions and becomes personal and client centered, as it should be.

Further, dually diagnosed individuals and their families should become aware of their right to addiction and mental health treatment when they are involved with law enforcement professionals and youth and family service personnel. The CSAT recommends training for judges and all law enforcement professionals so that individuals who have broken laws or who have parenting difficulties can be screened to ensure that they receive the most appropriate treatment. If dual-diagnosis issues are present, they need to be addressed by proper treatment and education.

The need for advocacy for better treatment for dually diagnosed individuals becomes glaringly clear when considering the statistics provided to me by my former employer at a psychosocial outpatient program in New Jersey, one of the states that provides the most effective treatment for dually diagnosed clients:

- The average Supplemental Security Income check for a dually diagnosed client is $585 per month, with a minimal amount per month in food stamps. For dually diagnosed clients who are unable to work and supplement this income, this amount of money barely covers living expenses.
- Social Security is stopping all SSI benefits and Medicaid for people who have an outstanding felony charge against them or are incarcerated.
- Dually diagnosed clients who are released from jail face long delays in having these benefits reinstated. For those who become violent when mentally unstable and/or using drugs, jail often is a recurring fact of life due to this lack of benefits.

STAYING WELL:
THE IMPORTANCE OF CONTINUING CARE

Clients who are stable on medication and sober have a strong need to receive outpatient services. Medicaid is now beginning to reduce the number of days they will allow for someone to attend partial care programs. Severely impaired clients whose partial care program had become their "family" now face portions of the week without a safe, educational environment due to reduced coverage. Education about mental illness, addiction, daily living skills, and medication needs to be ongoing and constant if clients are to avoid relapse.

In all states, treatment for dually diagnosed clients is strongly affected by the unwillingness of private insurance companies to fund adequate numbers of sessions for treatment issues to be thoroughly addressed. The CSAT suggests that advocacy needs to focus on educating insurance companies about the cost-effectiveness of providing thorough and comprehensive treatment so that dually diagnosed individuals may enter and remain in a continuum of care that would enable them to maintain wellness. Presently, managed care insurance may provide coverage for fewer than twelve sessions of outpatient treatment—clearly not enough time for the intense education and support needed by most dually diagnosed individuals. Consequently, individuals may constantly reenter treatment, need psychiatric hospitalization, or require inpatient addiction treatment.

Inpatient coverage for dually diagnosed clients has been reduced as well. Our current inpatient stays in detox of three to five days do not provide adequate opportunity for dually diagnosed clients to be free of substances and stable on medication. A period as long as twenty-one days in rehab (as portrayed in the vignettes you have read) is becoming increasingly unavailable to dually diagnosed clients in all states, yet it often takes at least this long for clients to receive an accurate diagnosis and medication that can begin to help.

State psychiatric hospitals in most states have some level of services for dually diagnosed clients, but they are not well funded. Further, they do not provide the consistent benefit of cross-trained staff who can address addiction needs in conjunction with mental health needs—one addiction counselor may have a caseload of as many as 200 people.

HOPE FOR THE FUTURE:
THE SEARCH FOR QUALITY OF LIFE

Getting and staying well are only parts of the battle faced by people who are dually diagnosed. It takes a long time to restore self-esteem and confidence after battling addiction and mental illness on an ongoing basis. Once people get beyond the daily struggle for stability and independence, they experience an increased desire for quality of life and the opportunity to set and reach goals. Many questions arise at this time as to what will constitute quality of life for individuals with a dual diagnosis, and housing is usually one of the first concerns.

Most states offer few options for safe housing for dually diagnosed clients. Many live with their families, environments that can include enablement, abuse, and other dysfunctions. Boarding homes are an option, but they often take all but a few dollars of a client's Social Security check and, in turn, provide an environment where drug and alcohol use may be rampant. Halfway houses in most states have become next to impossible for dually diagnosed individuals to enter, as such places often refuse clients who are on medication.

Quality of life for dually diagnosed clients is directly related to their ability to remain abstinent. If clients are able to have a good support system, careful medication monitoring, assistance in daily living skills and in maintaining relationships, and meaningful work, then quality of life can be quite satisfactory. However, too few dually diagnosed clients receive the empowerment they need to negotiate the system. Many have learning disabilities, are thought disordered, or are depressed. They need a system consisting of fewer steps that is easier for them to negotiate.

Thanks to well-known persons such as Tipper Gore, Betty Ford, Mary Tyler Moore, and many others who have gone public with their views on addiction and mental health issues, society's attitudes are changing for the better. We are coming to realize that addiction is a disease, not a moral issue. Advertisements on prime-time television publicize the help that is available for persons with serious mental illness. As a result of this public exposure the shame and secrecy regarding both of these diseases is gradually diminishing.

It is my hope that the stories in this book have touched your heart as they touched mine. Dually diagnosed people deserve our compassion. Their struggle deserves our understanding. Finally, their dignity, courage, and perseverance deserve our respect and our continuing advocacy.

Suggested Readings

Alcoholics Anonymous. *The Big Book,* Fourth Edition. New York: AA World Services, 2000. This is the primary recovery text for alcoholics and can be bought at most AA meetings.

Alcoholics Anonymous. *Living Sober.* New York: AA World Services, 1960. This book gives helpful advice for maintaining sobriety, one day at a time.

Alcoholics Anonymous. *Twelve Steps and Twelve Traditions.* New York: AA World Services, 1991. This book is used at "step" meetings of Alcoholics Anonymous and is helpful in explaining how AA maintains its principles and standards.

American Psychiatric Association. *Diagnostic and Statistical Manual of Mental Disorders,* Fourth Edition. Washington, DC: Author, 1994. This manual, used by psychiatrists but understandable to laypeople, is a reference for diagnosing mental illnesses.

Barnes, C. *A Program for You: A Guide to the Big Book's Design for Living.* New York: AA World Services, 1991. This book is helpful in teaching how knowledge of the twelve steps can promote change in one's life.

Beattie, M. *Codependent No More.* New York: Harper/Hazelden, 1987. This easy-to-read book is about how codependency affects family members of those who are addicted.

Black, C. *It Will Never Happen to Me.* New York: Ballantine Books, 1991. This highly readable book provides insight into family issues related to addiction.

Burns, D.D. *Feeling Good: The New Mood Therapy.* New York: Avon, 1980. This text shows how changing the way one thinks helps to combat depression.

Gorski, T. *Passages Through Recovery: An Action Plan for Preventing Relapse.* Center City, MN: Hazelden, 1989. This text gives instruction on ways of coping with addiction issues in early, middle, and late recovery.

Hazelden Foundation. *The Dual Disorders Recovery Book.* Center City, MN: Hazelden, 1993. This book gives specific, easy-to-follow guidelines for combining mental illness treatment with addiction treatment.

Kreisman, J.J. and Strauss, H. *I Hate You—Don't Leave Me: Understanding the Borderline Personality.* New York: Avon Books, 1989. This fascinating book describes behaviors that are reflected by people suffering from borderline personality disorder.

Mooney, A.J., Eisenberg, A., and Eisenberg, H. *The Recovery Book.* New York: Workman Publishing, 1992. This book answers common questions and concerns of recovering alcoholics and addicts.

Narcotics Anonymous, Fifth Edition. New York: Narcotics Anonymous Worldwide, 1988. This is the basic text used by most recovering people attending NA meetings.

Nilson, Mary Y. *When a Bough Breaks.* New York: Harper & Row, 1987. This book, combining documentary, fiction, and autobiography, dramatizes a family's experiences with a child's chemical dependency.

Torrey, E.F. *Surviving Schizophrenia: A Family Manual.* New York: Harper & Row, 1983. This is a comprehensive, easy-to-follow manual that answers commonly asked questions about living with schizophrenia.

Index

Addiction, as outward reach for inner
    peace, 95-96
Al-Anon, 5, 24
Alcoholics Anonymous (AA), 3
Anger, during treatment
    isolation, 88-89
    Marley's story, 84-88
    reasons for, 81-84

Children, reaction to parent's illness,
    17-18
Choices, 4
Counsel for Substance Abuse
    Treatment (CSAT), 115-116

Denial, 61-62
Depression/Anxiety Support Group, 4
Depressive and Manic Depressive
    Association (DMDA), 4
Dissociative identity disorder
    Arlene's story, 91-94
    described, 89-91
Double Trouble, 4
Dual diagnosis
    and family system
        Beverly's story, 6-9
        common scenarios, 2-3
        death of family member, 23-29
        effects of too much caretaking,
           10-17
        Eleanor's story, 25-29
        family as enemy, 17-23
        Jesús' story, 12-16
        Penny's story, 18-23
        role of family, 4-10

Dual diagnosis *(continued)*
    improving treatment options
        finding and receiving appropriate
           treatment, 113-115
        importance of continuing care,
           116-117
        need for advocacy, 115-116
        search for quality of life, 117-118
    misunderstandings about
        Allan's story, 71-76
        anger, 81-89
        Arlene's story, 91-94
        Craig's story, 63-68
        denial, 61-62
        dissociative identity disorder,
           89-94
        getting over on people, 76-81
        grandiosity, 69-76
        importance of acceptance, 62-63
        Josh's story, 78-81
        Marley's story, 84-88
        normal versus abnormal
           behavior, 63-68
    role of hope, empowerment, and
        spirituality in recovery
        Antonio's story, 97-100
        empowerment, 100-106
        Fred's story, 106-110
        hope, 97-100
        spirituality, 106-110
        Susan's story, 100-106

Empowerment
    importance of, 24-25
    in recovery of dually diagnosed
        clients, 97, 100-106

Family system, dual diagnosis and
  Beverly's story, 6-9
  common scenarios, 2-3
  death of family member, 23-29
  effects of too much caretaking,
    10-17
  Eleanor's story, 25-29
  family as enemy, 17-23
  Jesús' story, 12-16
  Penny's story, 18-23
  role of family, 4-10
Ford, Betty, 118

Gibran, Kahlil, 10
Gore, Tipper, 118
Grandiosity, 69-76
Group homes, 5
GROW, 4
Guilt, 5

Halfway houses, 5
Hero concept, 11-12
Home group, 3-4
Hope, in recovery of dually diagnosed
  clients, 96, 97-100

Life-giving, 25

Medication, 45, 58-59
Mood swings, 70-71
Moore, Mary Tyler, 118
Multiple personality disorder. *See*
    Dissociative identity disorder

Nar-Anon, 24
Narcotics Anonymous (NA), 3
National Alliance for the Mentally Ill
    (NAMI), 5

Parents of Bi-Polar Children, 4
Personality changes, 69-70
Personality disorder, 76-78
The Prophet (Gibran), 10

Reconnecting, 10-11
Resistance, to treatment. *See* Treatment
    resistance

Self Help Group Clearinghouse, 4
Shadow self, 90
Shame, 5
Spirituality, in recovery of dually
    diagnosed clients, 96, 106-110
Sponsors, 3
Stories
  dual diagnosis and family system
    Beverly, 6-9
    Eleanor, 25-29
    Jesús, 12-16
    Penny, 18-23
  misunderstandings about dual
    diagnosis
    Allan, 71-76
    Arlene, 91-94
    Craig, 63-68
    Josh, 78-81
    Marley, 84-88
  resistance to treatment
    Amanda, 40-45
    Candy, 48-52
    Melanie, 34-38
    Vincent, 54-58
  role of hope, empowerment, and
    spirituality in recovery
    Antonio, 97-100
    Fred, 106-110
    Susan, 100-106

Tough love, 1-2, 96
Treatment Improvement Protocol (TIP
    #9), 115

Order a copy of this book with this form or online at:
http://www.haworthpress.com/store/product.asp?sku=5111

ADDICTED AND MENTALLY ILL
Stories of Courage, Hope, and Empowerment

_____in hardbound at $34.95 ((ISBN: 0-7890-1885-3)

_____in softbound at $16.95 (ISBN: 0-7890-1886-1)

Or order online and use special offer code HEC25 in the shopping cart.

COST OF BOOKS_____

POSTAGE & HANDLING_____
(US: $4.00 for first book & $1.50
for each additional book)
(Outside US: $5.00 for first book
& $2.00 for each additional book)

SUBTOTAL_____

IN CANADA: ADD 7% GST_____

STATE TAX_____
(NJ, NY, OH, MN, CA, IL, IN, & SD residents,
add appropriate local sales tax)

FINAL TOTAL_____
(If paying in Canadian funds,
convert using the current
exchange rate, UNESCO
coupons welcome)

☐ **BILL ME LATER:** (Bill-me option is good on
US/Canada/Mexico orders only; not good to
jobbers, wholesalers, or subscription agencies.)
☐ Check here if billing address is different from
shipping address and attach purchase order and
billing address information.

Signature_____

☐ **PAYMENT ENCLOSED: $**_____

☐ **PLEASE CHARGE TO MY CREDIT CARD.**

☐ Visa ☐ MasterCard ☐ AmEx ☐ Discover
☐ Diner's Club ☐ Eurocard ☐ JCB

Account #_____

Exp. Date_____

Signature_____

Prices in US dollars and subject to change without notice.

NAME_____

INSTITUTION_____

ADDRESS_____

CITY_____

STATE/ZIP_____

COUNTRY_____ COUNTY (NY residents only)_____

TEL_____ FAX_____

E-MAIL_____

May we use your e-mail address for confirmations and other types of information? ☐ Yes ☐ No
We appreciate receiving your e-mail address and fax number. Haworth would like to e-mail or fax special
discount offers to you, as a preferred customer. **We will never share, rent, or exchange your e-mail address
or fax number.** We regard such actions as an invasion of your privacy.

Order From Your Local Bookstore or Directly From
The Haworth Press, Inc.
10 Alice Street, Binghamton, New York 13904-1580 • USA
TELEPHONE: 1-800-HAWORTH (1-800-429-6784) / Outside US/Canada: (607) 722-5857
FAX: 1-800-895-0582 / Outside US/Canada: (607) 771-0012
E-mailto: orders@haworthpress.com

For orders outside US and Canada, you may wish to order through your local
sales representative, distributor, or bookseller.
For information, see http://haworthpress.com/distributors

(Discounts are available for individual orders in US and Canada only, not booksellers/distributors.)
PLEASE PHOTOCOPY THIS FORM FOR YOUR PERSONAL USE.
http://www.HaworthPress.com   BOF04